# WHAT WOULD YOU LIKE TO DO?

The book takes the reader through Peter's life, the people he has met and the numerous ups and downs he has experienced in a way that is humorous, sometimes sad and frequently controversial.

This is not just an autobiography.

Peter talks about the women in his life, his views on management and, as a Christian, his philosophy of life. He uses many quotations which enriches the text and challenges the reader to relate to their own experiences. He documents what life was like not long past, but which in many ways is so different from today's age of hi-tech, mobile phones, personal computers and the internet.

Peter was born in 1944 and has lived through a period of history that has engineered technical advances and witnessed social changes and world globalization more than any other generation in history to date.

His working experience was in the financial services industry (mainly insurance underwriting) and he shows that, contrary to popular belief, it is a fascinating industry and not just a desk bound routine job.

Peter describes himself as an ordinary, normal and average person. He is not a celebrity but his experiences and his views on life show that he is far from just an ordinary man. By recording his memories and experiences Peter has created a history which future generations can explore and hopefully use so that their lives and the lives of future generations will be better.

Peter concludes by quoting an old friend of his, Andy Ripley, who played No. 8 for England and the British Lions at Rugby and who died in 2010 from prostate cancer:

> 'Dare we hope? We dare.
> Can we hope? We can.
> Should we hope? We must.
> We must, because to do otherwise is to waste the most
> precious of gifts, given so freely by God to all of us.
> So when we die, it will be with hope and it will be
> easy and our hearts will not be broken.'

All the proceeds and royalties from the sales of Peter's book are being donated to the Macmillan Cancer Support South East Appeal to build a support centre in Brighton for people and families in the South East of England affected by cancer and Peter is aiming to raise in excess of £20,000 for the Appeal.

This book is about his personal experience of living with cancer, so all views expressed are Peter's own and not those of Macmillan Cancer Support.

**WE ARE MACMILLAN.**
**CANCER SUPPORT**

# What would you like to do...?

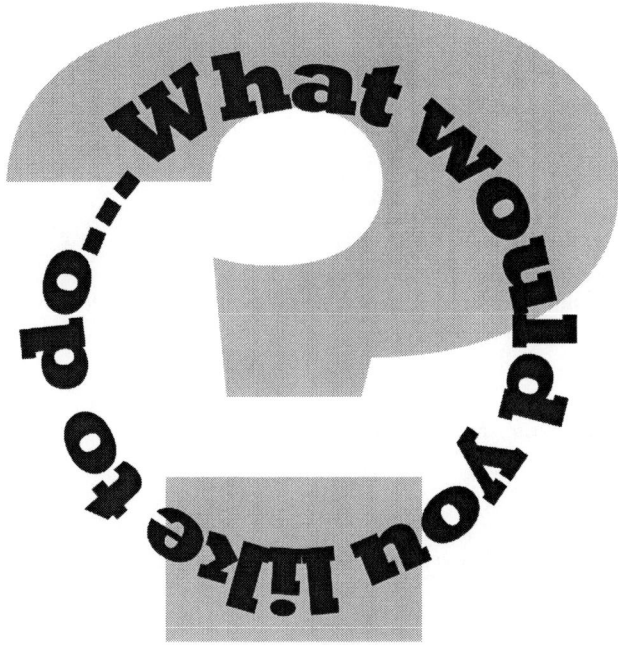

## The ultimate question

*Peter Sangster*

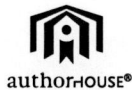

authorHOUSE®

*AuthorHouse™*
*1663 Liberty Drive*
*Bloomington, IN 47403*
*www.authorhouse.com*
*Phone: 1-800-839-8640*

*First published by AuthorHouse    08/27/2011*

*ISBN: 978-1-4567-9013-4 (sc)*
*ISBN: 978-1-4567-9014-1 (hc)*
*ISBN: 978-1-4567-9015-8 (ebk)*

*Printed in the United States of America*

# Foreword

In June 2010 I was diagnosed with an aggressive tumour on my right lung, and my consultant oncologist gave a prognosis of between 12 and 18 months. The first thing that my wife Linda asked me when we were driving home from the Conquest Hospital was:

WHAT WOULD YOU LIKE TO DO?

My first reaction was 'What a stupid question to ask—I have no idea what I want to do'.

This helped me to focus my brain on what I had just been told, and I decided two things.

The first was that, while I accepted the medical profession's diagnosis, with the help and expertise of the medical profession and my belief in the power of faith and prayer I would not give in but would fight my illness.

The second arose from my realisation that whenever someone dies, which we all will some day, all their memories and life experiences die with them unless they are recorded in some way. Therefore in my own humble way I decided that I should do something and record my own memories of life, for what it may be worth!

I am just an ordinary, normal and average person. The world is made up of millions of people just like me who may think that their lives are insignificant in the big picture. Our lives are not 'insignificant'; by recording our memories and experiences we create a history which future generations can explore and hopefully use so that their lives and the lives of future generations will be better.

In recent times a lot has been said about the National Health Service. I can only say that the speed of care and treatment, kindness and consideration that I have experienced from my own doctor and the East Sussex NHS Trust hospitals and staff have been exemplary. I include here the specialist nurses and teams supported by the MacMillan Cancer Support.

Linda, my wife, was a nurse for more than 35 years and cared for many sick people. She has also suffered first-hand from the trauma of coping personally with cancer. Her late husband died from cancer within less than six weeks of diagnosis. Soon afterwards, her son contracted Hodgkin's Disease but, thankfully, after radiotherapy treatment he seems to have completely recovered.

Linda and I feel immense appreciation and gratitude for the work which the MacMillan Cancer Support provide in the care and support of victims of cancer and their families.

All proceeds from my book will be donated to Macmillan Cancer Support.

This book is about my personal experience of living with cancer, so all views expressed are my own and not those of Macmillan Cancer Support.

*Peter Sangster*
*July 2011*

# WE ARE MACMILLAN.
## CANCER SUPPORT

# Acknowledgements

When I decided to write my book I discussed it with my close relatives and friends. It was their collective encouragement and cries of 'go for it' that spurred me on, and without their enthusiasm I do not think I would ever have started to write.

My greatest appreciation and thanks go to David Gordon, who has been a close friend for the past 18 years. David graduated in history from London University in 1963 before taking a post-graduate degree in teaching at Cambridge. His career was in the Merchant Navy, teaching cadets, until he retired in 1990. He then taught in learning disability centres for five years before spending some time as a relief teacher of primary school children. When I told David about my book, his enthusiasm was tempered by the warning that I could lose interest and never finish the project. I also knew that, never having written a book, my experience of writing was confined to business letters, memos and reports—not a style for easy reading.

David offered to be my 'don' and mentor and to critique my drafts. Not only did he do this, he also corrected my split infinitives, my boring repetitive use of words and long, one-sentence paragraphs, except for impact, and he was an inspiration in driving me onwards and not letting me relapse from my task. Without David's help I would not have completed this project.

I would also like to thank those friends and relatives, in particular my daughter Penny and my son Duncan, who helped me recall and correct my memories of events in my life.

To my lovely wife, Linda, I give my thanks. If she had not said to me:

WHAT WOULD YOU LIKE TO DO? I would not have written this book. There have been times when she wished I had not started, and on more than one occasion she has said that she will be happy when I finish and we can have a decent conversation again.

Finally, all those people whom I have never met but whom I have quoted in my book for their perceptions, which so often express so much more than I can in so few words.

I have tried to avoid this book being an autobiography, since Franklin P. Jones (1887–1929, President of the American Management Association) said:

An autobiography usually reveals nothing bad about its writer except his memory.

# Chapter 1
# THE QUESTION

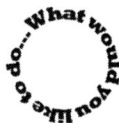

The Million Dollar Question if you were to be diagnosed with a terminal illness is:

WHAT WOULD YOU LIKE TO DO?

This is what most of us from time to time have asked ourselves in moments of private thought. Many of us have also asked or been asked this question as a party game or when we have confided it to our partner and/or friends after a good meal over a glass of port or with a mate over a pint of beer. The answers we came up with were nothing other than meaningless fancies and fantasies, such as getting absolutely 'rat-arsed' with the lads, going to exotic places we had not visited, or doing something that we had always dreamed about but which was totally out of the question or unrealisable, such as snogging Brigitte Bardot.

When I was told that I was faced with the reality of my situation, I realised that I had never answered this question properly in a dispassionate and constructive way, and I now realise that it is not only a stupid question to ask, but one that is totally impossible to answer unless you have to face this reality. How on earth can anyone possibly give an answer to it if they have no real understanding of the consequences facing them? It is only when you are actually told that you have a terminal illness, and you fully accept and understand what that means, that you realise the abject stupidity of this question! My advice is never to ask it either of yourself or of others, unless you are taking part in a silly fantasy party game like Consequences or Charades. To take such a question seriously is at best a total waste of time and at worst a way to depress yourself and become a hypochondriac for the rest of your life.

Don't get me wrong; it is good to have dreams. It is ambition based on dreams that drives us on and spurs us to achieve great things. A complacent acceptance of one's lot, with no dreams, is a recipe for an unhappy and unfulfilled life.

I have been a Christian believer from the age of nine, when I was a choirboy at St John's Church, Kenilworth. Or maybe my faith was implanted earlier, at the age of seven, when I was made to attend Sunday School, which I hated, and then joined the choir to escape the boredom of 'school again on Sundays'. All through my life, admittedly with varying degrees of commitment to prayer and worship, I have never lost or doubted this belief. Therefore my first thought was that death does not frighten me. Death is a happy occasion for the 'victim'; it is those who are left who are unhappy—but they shouldn't be!

I am probably no different from most people. I grew up through childhood, youth, early manhood and almost into middle age believing that I was indestructible and that death was something that only ever happened to other people. It was when I was 37, with a good job (with the inevitable big mortgage), happily married with two children aged eight and ten, and my father died of pneumonia following several uncomfortable years suffering from emphysema, that it dawned on me that life was in fact finite and that one day I also would actually die as well.

Following Dad's death, for the first time in my life I made a very serious attempt to stop smoking—one of numerous similar, failed attempts ever since. It is probably because of my failure to take due heed of all the medical evidence and advice that I have now been diagnosed with lung cancer. While I cannot be certain, medical evidence is that if I had stopped smoking I would probably not now be faced with the question WHAT WOULD YOU LIKE TO DO? However, it is not my intention to lecture anyone about the risks of smoking. As a smoker, the thing I hated most was all those 'boring farts' who had given up smoking banging on at me about giving it up. I also especially dislike the goody-goody 'I've never smoked' people who have not been so unfortunate as to have become hooked on what, as my 'never smoked' consultant oncologist Tim Sevitt told me, is now recognised by the medical profession as a drug more addictive than heroin.

The most wonderful thing about Christian belief and faith is that God gave us free will to make our own decisions, and that is what makes life and living so rich, diverse, dynamic, fun, most of the time wonderful, sometimes sad and too often evil—like getting hooked on nicotine! Carry on and make your own decisions, so long as you are content to accept the possible consequences, and good luck.

As I start to write my book, I have also started my chemotherapy treatment, not knowing exactly what the future holds for me. While doing so I reflect back over my life and I now realise that this question WHAT WOULD YOU LIKE TO DO? had in fact cropped up many times and had been answered in many different ways before, in fact whenever I reached a crossroad in my life. I now also realise that the decisions that I made and actions that I took on each occasion were answering this question, WHAT WOULD YOU LIKE TO DO? Sometimes the answer was an impulse, sometimes a result of serious consideration of material issues such as money, career prospects or other very selfish reasons. Just occasionally, the answer was for purer motives, driven by my Christian belief and ethics. What is most startling is the realisation that the decisions have not just determined what happened next in my life, but invariably resulted in meeting new people and making new friends, all of whom have themselves influenced the development of my character, opinions and behaviour and helped form the sort of person that I now am.

Two things happened when I was faced with the fact that I had a terminal illness.

First, I took this news, and a full realisation of the consequences, on board immediately, and 'in a flash' I knew the answer to WHAT WOULD YOU LIKE TO DO? The answer is very simple, and I will explain what it is, but only after I have been able to document my life experiences fully. I will try to explain all this over the following chapters of my book, as I take you through some of these life experiences and the people who have influenced me and formed me into the person that I am, whether you like it or not!

Second, I was angry. Not because of the realisation that my life expectancy was finite and I was going to die, but because I felt I was letting other people down.

It may seem a little strange that I, a Christian, could agree with an atheist, Christopher Hitchens, an author and essayist who was diagnosed with cancer of the oesophagus about the same time that I was diagnosed. In an interview with Jeremy Paxman in November 2010 he expressed this far better than I could.

> I have to sit passively every few weeks and have a huge dose of kill or cure venom put straight into my veins, and then follow that up with other poisons too. You feel as if you're drowning in passivity and being assaulted by something that

has a horrible persistence, that's working on you while you are asleep. I feel a sense of waste about it because I'm not ready. I feel a sense of betrayal to my family and even to some of my friends who would miss me. I am not scared of death, however I am frightened of a 'sordid' or 'squalid' death. My main fear is of being incapacitated or imbecilic at the end. That, of course, is not something to be afraid of—it's something to be terrified of.

The other thing that I ask you to reflect on as you read my book is your own experiences of life and its trials and tribulations and how they have affected you.

Stephen Covey, an American who lectures in human behaviour, expounds his '90/10' Principle, which states that ten per cent of life is made up of what happens to you, but ninety per cent of life is decided by how you react to that ten per cent. He goes on to illustrate this very lucidly in everyday situations.

Let's take an example. You are eating your breakfast with your family. Your daughter knocks over a cup of coffee on to your business shirt. You have no control over what has happened. What happens next will be determined by how you react. You curse. You harshly scold your daughter for knocking the cup over. She breaks down in tears. After scolding her, you turn to your spouse and criticize her for placing the cup too close to the edge of the table. A short verbal battle follows. You storm upstairs and change your shirt. Back downstairs, you find your daughter has been too busy crying to finish her breakfast and get ready for school. She misses the bus. Your spouse must leave immediately for work. You rush to the car and drive your daughter to school. Because you are late, you drive at 40mph in a 30mph speed limit. After a 15-minute delay and throwing the £60 fine away, you arrive at school. Your daughter runs into the building without saying goodbye. After arriving at the office 20 minutes late, you find you forgot your briefcase. Your day has started terribly. As it continues, it seems to get worse and worse. You look forward to coming home. When you arrive home you find a small wedge in your relationship with your spouse and daughter. Why? Because of how you reacted in the morning. Why did you have a bad day? A) Did the coffee cause it? B) Did your daughter cause it? C) Did the policeman cause it? D) Did you cause it? The answer is D. You had no control over what happened with the coffee. How you reacted in those five seconds is what caused your bad day.

Here is what should have happened. Coffee splashes over you. Your daughter is about to cry. You say gently 'It's OK, Honey, you just need to be more careful next time'. Grabbing a towel you rush upstairs. After grabbing a new shirt and your briefcase, you come back down in time to look through the window and see your child getting on the bus. She turns and waves. You arrive five minutes early and cheerfully greet your staff. Your boss comments on how good a day you are having. Notice the difference?

Both started the same way. Both ended different. Why? Because of how you REACTED. You really do not have control over 10% of what happens. The other 90% of what happens will be determined by your reaction to that 10%.

I have had my fair share of ups and downs, and yet somehow seem to have managed to come through them and emerged the better in the long run, but maybe I, as perhaps you, would have coped better if I had learned Stephen's 90/10 Principle sooner and applied it in my life more often.

## Chapter 2
# EARLY YEARS

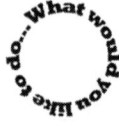

My father was born in Aberdeen in 1906. His father was a confectioner and baker. He had three brothers, one of whom died soon after birth, another in early childhood from diphtheria and the other at the age of 18 in a lift-shaft accident. My father was the only one to survive to adulthood. My mother was born in Dewsbury. Her father and his elder brother were brought up by their Uncle Oliver from early childhood, after their father emigrated to Australia, never to be seen or heard of again, and their mother died soon after, reputably of a 'broken heart'. My grandfather was a technical draughtsman and worked most of his life in local government. So my ancestry was not exceptional—they were just ordinary, good people.

So it is. The world in which we live is made up of millions of such ordinary, good people. Very few in their lifetime become famous or have an exceptional talent by which they are remembered by more than a handful of people. Even if they are famous, it is inevitably only in a very narrow field or profession. Unless a biography is written of someone's life, when they die all their memories and their life experiences and views of life are lost with them forever. This is why I am writing this book. It is not for self-gratification, although it gives me some pleasure to achieve a long-held ambition. I hope that someone, some time in the future, will enjoy reading about Peter Sangster's ordinary life and the ramblings of an ordinary person, and either find in it interesting information about their ancestry, or enjoy reading about my memories and understanding of what life was like in my times and relate this to their own life experiences.

Lewis Grizzard, an American writer and humourist, once said:

Life is a sexually transmitted terminal disease.

How relevant this is. Regardless of whether or not a person has faith or is indifferent, it is a historical fact that you were born and that you have already experienced many things, both good and bad. The other fact is that at some time in the future you will die.

I was born on 6th January 1944, half Scottish and half Yorkshire by ancestry. Someone once defined a Yorkshireman as 'a Scotsman with the generosity squeezed out of him'. I always found that amusing, despite my breeding. Like most, I have no recollection of the first two years or so of my life, so have no memories of the end of the Second World War. My sister, Brenda, remembers more about life in those days and has written the following account of her own memories, entitled *Then and Now*.

My grandfather died in 1947 after a short illness. What a shock he would have if he came alive again today!

He never saw television. He loved Gilbert and Sullivan music and had records of all the operas, which he played on a wind-up gramophone. He would also listen to the wireless and I remember that we all had to keep quiet when the news was on—a habit formed during the war years.

He walked to the village shops every day to get his cigarettes, which he smoked heavily, as did most people in those days. My grandmother would also visit the shops every day, buying fresh food. There were no fridges in the house, just a larder with a marble slab and a bucket of cold water outside in the shade to stand the milk in to prevent it going sour. This was delivered daily by the milkman in a horse and carriage. Groceries like sugar, flour, butter and biscuits, etc. were all weighed by an assistant in the shop and packed into either greaseproof paper or paper bags. These were then burnt, either on the kitchen fire or on a bonfire in the garden—no need for recycling. No plastic bags and definitely a lot less wastage. There were no supermarkets, so the grocer, the butcher, the baker, the newsagent, etc., all had to be visited individually.

Monday was washday and Granddad would light the boiler in the wash house at the bottom of the garden, and then Granny would spend all morning washing the clothes by hand and boiling the white cottons, adding a dolly blue to add to the whiteness. She would then turn the handle on a large mangle to get excess water out of each article before hanging them on a line in the garden or, if inclement, on a rack above the kitchen fire. This was hoisted up and down with a pulley. On Tuesday the ironing would be done with an iron which was heated on the fire. No detergents, just soap, no washing machines, tumble driers or electric irons.

On Wednesday the house was cleaned—carpets were lifted and taken outside to be beaten with a wicker carpet beater as they hung on the washing line. This beating got all the dust out. The floors were then brushed and mopped before the carpets were replaced. The furniture was dusted and polished with wax until it shone and smelt clean and fresh. No vacuum cleaners or fitted carpets, and carbolic soap to use to scrub the floor on hands and knees with a scrubbing brush.

The fireplace was cleaned out regularly and blackened. There were ovens on either side of the fire and hotplates which could be moved over the fire to boil the kettle or saucepans. We all huddled round the fire in winter—no central heating. Upstairs was so cold. The beds had feather mattresses, lots of woolly blankets and a big eiderdown on top, so once in bed it was very cosy. The double beds had a bolster with two feather pillows on top. A warming pan was sometimes used to warm the cold cotton sheets. This was a pan and lid with a long handle, into which hot coals from the fire were put in the pan and it was taken upstairs and rubbed around the bed. The hot water bottles were made of pottery and were most uncomfortable. No electric blankets or warm duvets.

If my grandparents wanted to get in touch with family or friends they would either post a letter or, if urgent, send a telegram, which would be delivered by a boy on a bike in a few hours, or maybe they would use the nearest telephone box. Not many people had a telephone at home, and of course there were no mobile phones or computers.

My grandparents never went abroad. Their holidays were always taken the first two weeks of September at a hotel in Scarborough. They went by train as they did not own a car and neither of them ever drove. They saved for everything they needed and wouldn't dream of getting into debt. There were certainly no credit cards or hire purchase, just pawnbrokers in the towns for anyone desperate enough to use them.

For relaxation my grandfather would go to the bowls club or watch the local cricket team, and would listen avidly to the wireless to the results of county and test matches, especially if his beloved Yorkshire were playing. In the evenings they would play cards and several times a week go to a whist drive in the village. Granddad had an allotment as well as a very pretty garden, and if the milkman's horse left its droppings near his house would always be out with a shovel to place the manure on his prize roses.

Granny never wore make-up as Granddad didn't approve of it. My mother told me that when she started going out for dates she would have to put her make-up on after she left the house and take it off before getting home. He was so strict about this and often quoted 'Little dabs of powder, little pots of paint make a little lady really what she ain't'.

How times have changed in sixty odd years! Have they changed for the better? I'm not so sure, life was so much simpler in those days, but they did work hard. We have so much these days and lots of people try to 'keep up with the neighbours' and seem so discontented with life. I'm glad, however, that I have lived to see the changes and am pleased that I can't remember the worries of the last two world wars.

I wonder what changes the next sixty years will bring and what our grandchildren will remember about us!

My first recollections were when we lived in Mumbles in South Wales. My father, having been de-mobbed after the war from the RAF, resumed his business career in insurance and was posted to work in the company's Swansea branch. I always remember my mother telling me that those were the happiest years of her life. The war was over and, although times were difficult with rationing and restrictions placed on the availability of food and luxuries, living as a family together for the first time made her very happy. She loved Mumbles, and I remember going down to the beach when the tide was out, collecting cockles with my mother's parents, who often came to stay with us. Granddad was a bundle of fun. Once in April, after a shower of rain, the sunshine came out and we stood under a laburnum tree in the garden. Granddad shook it and we all got soaked and could not stop laughing. The other thing I remember was how in those days of rationing he used to save up his butter ration and then blow it all in one breakfast sitting by ladling it thick on his toast, saying he loved to feel his teeth sinking into it. How I resemble Granddad, although I don't have to save up my butter rations to do it today. Granddad died when I was only three, and sadly I was far too young to realise the significance of this. I would like to have known him better. *C'est la vie ou la mort.*

My grandmother lived to the good old age of 84, and right up to the end, every evening she would go on the bus to whist drives. She was also a heavy smoker who could best be described as 'fag-ash Lill' since cigarette ash was constantly spilt down the front of her dress. My father's mother suffered from arthritis, and she had very swollen and painful knees. As a result, Granny and Granddad rarely travelled far from their home in Southport, so the only times we saw them were when we went to visit, usually at Easter. Granny was quite crippled, and I suspect that she suffered from rheumatoid arthritis, which I have had for the past 15 years. I can vouch for the fact that swollen knees can be very painful and debilitating. In those days knowledge and medication were not as available as they are today. I heard on a Radio 4 programme recently that a doctor had discovered that RA has a hereditary link, but that the disease often skips a generation. So I can thank Granny Sangster for my RA. Granny was also a bit of a Mrs Malaprop, and in particular I remember that she used to tell us that she had been poorly and the doctor had given her 'penny shilling'. Another one was that she used to call rhododendrons 'rosiedondrons'. Whenever you tried to correct her she would just say 'Och, that's what they call it in Scotland'—end of discussion. She was a bit of a stickler, and on another occasion, when they were about 70 years old, she sent Granddad out to sell his 15-year-old Ford motor car and give up driving. Granddad came back three hours later, still with the car. In the back of the car was their first television (black and white, of course). Being a bit deaf, he proceeded to put it on at full volume and ignored Granny's ranting and raving about how irresponsible he was.

My sister, Brenda, was nearly five years older than me and used to play some rather nasty tricks on me. Once when we were in a café I pointed at a pot of yellow stuff on the table and asked what it was. Brenda said it was called mustard and was absolutely delicious. She told me to put my finger in and have a lick. I did. I have never touched Coleman's English Mustard again. I also remember asking her for a piggyback, and she told me to stand on the step and jump on her back. I did. She moved away and the result was that I knocked in my front teeth and there was a lot of blood and tears. For the next few years I had a gaping chasm in the front of my mouth, and Mother frequently recalled the time when two ladies saw me and one said 'Look at that little boy with long eyelashes and no teeth', and then proceeded to roar with laughter. I did not see the funny side of this story!

Even as a toddler, apparently, I enjoyed chatting up the ladies. One of our neighbours in Mumbles was a Mrs Marbett, and her husband had a big car. One day when I popped in to see her she was cooking pancakes in a frying pan, and it is reputed that I said to her 'You may have the biggest car in the road but my mum has the biggest frying pan'.

When I was about five years old my father was asked to stand in as relief manager of his company's Stoke on Trent office, following the unexpected death of the incumbent. I suspect that this was a career opportunity too good to turn down, so, despite the happy time in South Wales, we moved to Trentham, where we lived for a year.

My parents sent me to my first school in Trentham, which was called Spot House. Damn, now I have gone and exposed the answer to one of my secret questions for my email address. What the hell! If, as I have already found to my inconvenience, a hacker wants to break in and steal my emails, they have far more sophisticated ways of doing it than by knowing the name of my first school.

At Spot House I remember I was very happy and, as it was one of the old-fashioned boys' prep schools, I very quickly learned cursive ('proper joined-up') handwriting. Soon after, Father was asked to move to Coventry and open a brand-new office for the company and develop business in the Midlands. We bought a house in the suburbs of Coventry. I then went to Styvechale School, a local mixed primary school which was not only a new school but also grossly over-crowded, with class sizes of up to 40. I was forbidden to continue with writing in joined-up letters and made to go backwards to be at the same level as the other kids. I have since believed that one of the biggest problems of the state education system is the great danger that pupils can be dragged down to the lowest common level rather than being encouraged to aspire to higher standards. I know that in recent years the education system has improved greatly, but I mention this (and hasten to add that I am not a hard right-wing part of the so-called 'privileged classes') for any parents who share my concern. The only sound solution seems to me to send your children to a private fee-paying school. It is worth the sacrifice and hardship if you can, and the best way in your life is to spend your money investing in the future generation, especially your own blood.

My wife, Alli, and I experienced this same problem with our son, Duncan. At a secondary modern school in East Grinstead where our daughter was doing very well, Duncan was being dragged down by his peers. We were faced with that inevitable question, WHAT WOULD YOU LIKE TO DO about it? Fortunately, when he was 13 I had a career move from Sussex to the North West and we were able to put enough cash on one side to afford to send him to Birkenhead School as a fee-paying pupil. It did not raise Duncan's academic ability since, thanks to his mum and dad, he does not have the right genes for that, but it did help him. From being a no-chancer he got reasonable GCSEs and went on to take A Levels. It also developed his character and other talents which have stood him in good stead throughout his life and will continue to do so. Duncan on many occasions said to Alli and me that, of all the things that we ever did for him, paying for him to go to Birkenhead School was the best.

I am sad to say that at Styvechale I got into some bad company, and one day when I was only eight, and soon before November 5th, other boys dared me to pinch some fireworks from a nearby shop. Because I had never stolen anything before I was a total amateur, and so was caught red-handed. I can definitely say from this experience that the fear of being caught is a far greater deterrent to crime than the punishment is. I was given a severe telling-off by a policeman and sent home. Nothing else happened, and to this day I do not know whether the police told my parents, but to me it was a lesson which I have never forgotten. I have never since even been tempted to fiddle my expenses, unlike some! The next year I fell over, having been pushed by one of the other boys while playing on the common in front of our house, and suffered a compound fracture of my right elbow. That was when kids learned by experiencing danger and risk as part of growing up. We used to do things like climbing trees, and playing conkers and British Bulldogs in the school playground. No-one had heard of risk assessment or health and safety. I spent three weeks in hospital and had two operations. This was a changing moment in my life. I was so fascinated by the hospital, the doctors and the nurses that I decided that I wanted to be a doctor when I grew up. This ambition remained with me for the next ten years. Soon after I came out of hospital my parents took my sister and me on holiday for two weeks to Paignton, and as we arrived I came out in spots and was diagnosed with chickenpox. I was confined for the entire two weeks to the hotel bedroom, itching like mad, even using Mother's knitting needles to stick underneath the plaster on my right arm to scratch hidden spots. I also remember that it poured with rain for virtually the whole time, so it was not the best holiday we ever had.

By now it was becoming obvious to my parents that, not only was I in the bottom 10th percentile at school, but my chances of passing the 11-plus were nil and I would be faced with going to one of the new comprehensive schools in Coventry. From some poor reports about the success of the new comprehensive education system, my parents were very concerned, and my father paid for me to have some private lessons in Maths and English, as a result of which I was just able to scrape through the entrance examination for King Henry VIII School Coventry and was accepted as a fee-paying pupil. It was about the same time that my father, in a fit of pique over the rude behaviour of one of the little brats who lived next door to us and was totally undisciplined by his parents, smacked the boy. The boy's parents reported this to the police, claiming that my father had assaulted their son. Fortunately the police decided not to take any action, but imagine the disgrace we would have suffered as a family if he had been prosecuted! This was in the 'good-old-bad-old' days of the mid-1950s, when reasonable corporal punishment to correct children's behaviour was considered acceptable. I remember that our form master at school used to slipper us if we transgressed, and there were several occasions when I was made to bend over in front of the whole class, including girls (who were not slippered but smacked on the hand). On one occasion I was a bit upset because I was slippered when the transgression was not my fault but that of one of the other boys. When I got home and complained to my father about it he sent me to bed early for complaining and not accepting my punishment like a man.

Soon after this we moved house to Kenilworth and I started at King Henry VIII.

# Chapter 3
# THE TEENS

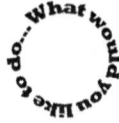

King Henry VIII School was a private school in the Direct Grant Grammar School system, taking in those who had excelled in their 11-plus (paid for by the local authority) and others like me who had passed the entrance examination as fee-paying pupils. It therefore had a wide cross-section of pupils from all backgrounds. I really enjoyed King Henry VIII, especially the tuckshop and rugby. I took a real shine to the sciences, especially biology and chemistry, which spurred me on further in my ambition to be a doctor. The school operated a method of streaming in each academic year. W.B. Yeats once said:

> Education is not the filling of a bucket, but the lighting of a fire.

So it was at King Henry VIII; teaching was inspiring, and pupils were challenged and encouraged to achieve and improve themselves. I responded to this.

I started in form 2E (the bottom form in the first year, the top form being 2A) and, because of my class work and end of year examination results, I progressed steadily each year, going up into 3D, then 4C and in the fourth year to Lower 5B. In the third year, we were allowed to select preferred subjects to enable each boy to start to specialise his education, but English Language and Maths were compulsory, as was R.I. I, wanting to specialise in the three sciences, had to drop two other subjects but had to continue with at least one language. The only modern language we had studied so far was French, and I was not very good at this, so the thought of German or Spanish was a non-starter. Because I still wanted to pursue a career in medicine I decided to drop French and continue with Latin. The added advantage of this was that, because there were set books which involved learning and understanding Roman history, I could also drop History as a subject.

I hated History, first because I could not see the point of having to learn about kings and queens and the dates of their reigns and viewed it as a subject which, unlike other subjects, was not dynamic but 'fixed', allowing no opportunity, as the sciences did, for research and new discovery. Later in life, having acquired an interest in military history, I realised how naive my views were. History by its nature is recording facts. Facts cannot be changed, but they can be re-interpreted on the basis of new evidence discovered. Lessons can be learned to help all of us to try to change life today and tomorrow and hopefully make the world in which we live a better place in the future. It seems to me a great pity that some politicians, not just ours but world-wide, far too often seem to ignore the lessons which history offers and continue to make what I believe are flawed decisions. At the time of writing in 2010 Afghanistan comes to my mind. No doubt when today and tomorrow become history, history will determine whether the politicians or I were right!

During these early years at King Henry VIII the changes brought on by puberty also had an effect on me. I was a later developer than some of my peers, some of whom even in the first year were showing the physical signs of manhood. These hormonal changes in an all-male environment, and the inevitable frustrations experienced in some, led to a tendency towards homosexual behaviour which I found totally distasteful. We now live in a more open and tolerant society, but even to this day I find it hard to see overt 'gay' behaviour as acceptable, and it is certainly not compatible with my own Christian beliefs. I put the word 'gay' in inverted commas because the English language is also a changing and dynamic subject, and to me this is an example of the worst debasement of what used to be a beautiful word. I fully understand that things have changed and that homosexuality is now fully acceptable in today's society, but as far as I am concerned, those of you who want to, please keep it to yourselves in private and do not expose it to me. I am very relaxed about being alongside people who are homosexual and even have friends who are homosexual, as I am with black, coloured and ethnic races and people with different creeds, but heterosexuals and others do not march through Brighton once a year exposing their private lives to everyone!

In 1957, the company that my father worked for was taken over, and then soon after the new group was acquired by the Sun Alliance Group (now RSA) and, as part of the re-organisation and merging of branch offices which inevitably takes place, Father was offered a choice of two very good positions: either inspector for London based in the City or chief inspector for the North West based in Liverpool.

Father had no hesitation in taking the post in Liverpool. And so it was that, having progressed at King Henry VIII to Lower 5B and just as my GCE O Level year was about to start, I was faced with a move of school. My father, with the assistance of the headmaster at King Henry VIII, secured a place for me at Merchant Taylors School Crosby (MTS), another Direct Grant School, but, as MTS had some boarders, it included Saturday school and games afternoon (as well as sport on Wednesday afternoon) which I found a relief since I did not know what I would have otherwise done on Saturdays. Whether it was a glowing report from the King Henry VIII headmaster or just the fact that the only form with a vacancy was Upper V Language (probably the latter), I started my O level year not only with a totally different syllabus (including different set books for Latin) and a different examining body, but also had to take General Science instead of the three separate sciences. I was also told that I had to take a modern language. I chose French, because I had studied it for three years, but had almost forgotten all but *oui* and *non*, and settled into a totally new environment and making new friends. Not the sort of situation I would recommend you subject your children to unless it is unavoidable, but I coped remarkably well.

Maybe it is because of the nature of the Scouser, but I found all my new classroom mates very friendly and I soon settled in and was able to continue my extra-curricular passion for singing in a church choir, now as a fully blown tenor. Gerald Brown was a new school colleague and his father was choirmaster at St Michael's Blundellsands. Gerald became one of my closest friends for the next 15 years. The church choir also used to stand in for the Liverpool Cathedral choir in August; to sing in such a wonderful place for acoustics was a real experience and privilege. Gerald also organised a youth choir which, apart from being my first close contact exposure to girls for many years, was extremely great fun. On Saturday afternoon when sports was cancelled I, with some of my school friends, would go to Anfield and stand in the Kop cheering Liverpool (who were then still in the old second football division) so my life-long support of the boys in red was not founded on the fact that they were a successful team. Also, on some Saturday nights we would go into Liverpool centre, and in Matthew Street there was a club called the Cavern where we would go to watch trad jazz (the likes of Humphrey Littleton, Chris Barber and Acker Bilk). The Cavern was not licensed and during the break we used to go to a pub in Matthew Street while an unknown group called the Beatles played to a fairly thin audience!

I recall little of the masters who taught me at school. At King Henry VIII I only really remember Mr Crocker, who was our Chemistry master and so inspiring in his teaching that he is hard ever to forget. At MTS, N.E.J. Wiley was a formidable man. His looks were cadaverous and as deputy head master he had the authority (and regularly used any opportunity to exercise it) to cane boys, but he really drummed the classics into us—particularly, in my case, Latin. Sadly, I suspect that his sort is one of past history. The other was a young Maths master (who struck me so much that I now cannot remember his name!) but he arrived at MTS straight from Cambridge for his first teaching post. He had left King Henry VIII only just before I started in my first year there, and I remember observing with amusement that he was still very spotty and squirted his face with Germaline to try and cover up the bad ones.

Initially, because Mum and Dad had not yet bought a house and moved, I stayed for the first term with my Granny, who lived in Crosby. Granny went out to her whist drive every evening and I set out to do as much prep (homework) as I could to catch up on French and to learn the new Latin set books. I did not spend a great deal of effort on General Science since I already knew most of the syllabus, having previously taken the three sciences separately. Because of my dislike of language subjects, I was amazed that somehow I actually managed to pass French and Latin O level. The French I put down to the oral examination, which most of my colleagues dreaded but I relished. I remember going into the room to be faced with two rather strict-looking elderly ladies and going straight up to them with my hand outstretched, saying '*Bonjour, Mesdames, je suis Pierre. Comment allez vous?*'. People who know me well and that sometimes I can be bold, even a bit outrageous, will believe that I did this. I think that the two ladies were so taken aback that, whatever happened thereafter, they felt they could not fail me!

I did reasonably well in other subjects, with 90% in General Science, but I failed English Language. It then took me a further two attempts while in the VIth form to pass this irritating subject—how can anyone fail in his mother tongue? I understand that Winston Churchill was also a duff at English and once said that at Harrow School he had been made to retake the same year syllabus three times, to which he attributed his incredible command of our lovely language.

Maybe I am in good company. My main problem was that the essay carried a substantial number of marks and I was not a creative or flowery sort of writer and the stupid subjects they gave us such as A Hot Summer's Day or My Favourite Pet were a complete turn-off for me. Some sad old boy when he died had left the school a legacy for all VIth formers for an essay prize, and at the end of each Lent term we were given subjects and on the first morning back for Summer term we were put in exam conditions for two hours and made to write an essay on one of the subjects. The difference from O level English exams was that we were given interesting subjects such as The Future Problem of World Food Shortage. In the Lower VIth my essay was commended, and in the second year I won the prize, despite the fact that I was the only boy who still had not yet passed O level English! An English master took me to one side and said 'Sangster, use more exciting words in your essays such as "unembellished"', so I trawled the OED for such words to use and at my third attempt I passed!

Because of my pass mark in General Science (I guess equivalent to grade A today) I was allowed to go into Lower VIth (Biology) and study Biology, Chemistry and Physics for A Level, so I was back on track to achieve my ambition to study medicine at university and become a doctor. At MTS, the VIth form syllabus included compulsory lectures in cultural subjects which were not part of our mainstream studying but which were, nevertheless, considered important in the process of continuing a balanced education to widen understanding. In particular I remember the cultural periods for Maths and R.I. In Maths we learned about statistical methods and how to apply the subject to real-life situations, which has held me in good stead all my life. Our R.I. master was a C of E priest but he taught us the basics of all major religions of the world other than Christianity. Not only did I find this fascinating, since it gave me an insight into other beliefs and cultures, but in a roundabout way it served to further strengthen my belief that God does exist and that Christ was in fact the Son of God.

By the time I started at MTS I had developed physically and caught up with my earlier peers, and I really enjoyed sports, particularly rugby. However, not having a natural ball sense, I played in the forwards at rugby, where you can play a reasonable game while hardly ever having to touch the ball except in close contact. I did not shine at cricket and that hard little ball really hurt when it hit you—I did not mind getting hurt but in cricket, unlike rugby, you could not easily get your own back! In order to get out of playing cricket I joined the rowing club, which meant an all-year-round commitment, so I was then able to play rugby only during the last two years, in the annual house matches. Rowing, I soon learned, was about the most athletic sport, in that you use more muscles in your body than in any other sport. Being part of a crew, when you became exhausted you could not ease off, and it also taught me how to go through the pain barrier and greatly developed my character and sense of team spirit.

The other passion of mine at MTS was the Combined Cadet Force. The military life and the discipline really appealed to me, and I always looked forward to the last two periods on Tuesday and Thursday afternoons, and the field days and the pomp of the parades on Armistice Day and our annual inspections. Once we had passed our basic training we could apply to transfer to the Navy or RAF sections, but I preferred to continue to be a 'brown job'. I joined the band and learned (rather badly) to play the bugle and drums, and in the summer holidays I went on a two-week REME course at Bordon in Hampshire, learning how to service Land Rovers, to fault-find and repair when a vehicle had broken down. By the time I left school I had risen to the dizzy rank of Colour Sergeant and was determined that I would pursue the Army in some way, either in the university OTC or in the TA.

While at MTS I had three really good pals, each of whom in his different way left an impact on my life. I have already mentioned Gerald Brown. Gerald was a brilliant musician and, apart from being a dynamic and enthusiastic person (although, as artistic people often are, he was also a temperamental character), he had a fantastic sense of humour and was a great mate. It is thanks to Gerald that I developed the love of four-part choral singing which I still enjoy today. I lost contact with Gerald when I moved south in 1969, and heard with sadness that he died soon after my father in 1980 from a massive heart attack when driving home from work one evening. I will always remember Gerald, and the fun and the love of choral music that he gave to me.

The second pal was Alan Walker (Curlie). Curlie and I were in the Sixth Form Biology stream and carried out a lot of 'experiments' together. For example, in those days we bred white rats in the bio lab and killed them humanely with chloroform before dissecting them as part of our A Level practical examination syllabus. Often this meant blood everywhere, but it made taking our final exam easy because the rats provided by the examining board were preserved in formic acid and quite dry! Curlie was more academic than me and, although only five foot six inches, was also very athletic and muscular, and we were in the rowing club together. I had great difficulty in matching his physical abilities, as well as his superior academic prowess. We were in these ways a bit of opposites, but we both had a passion for jazz—initially trad but later modern—and were lucky enough to see Dave Brubeck live in concert in Liverpool.

During the summer of 1962 while we were awaiting our A Level results Curlie and I earned some cash on the casual labour at Liverpool docks. This was a real experience. Casual labour on Liverpool docks meant that you had to get a 'green card' from the employment exchange and could turn up in what was called The Pens on the docks shouting 'job, job, job' and banging your green card. The supervisors would then select a gang to unload a shipment of cargo. If you were not selected you would go to one of the many dock road pubs and wait for the next opportunity to seek a job again. Curlie and I, having got a couple of jobs and earned a bit of cash, then hitch-hiked up the A6 (no M6 in those days) to the Lake District and spent four weeks camping and rock climbing. This was the first time that I experienced freedom from parents, family life and a protected environment and learned how to cope with having to look after myself. It was a great holiday. When we left school Curlie and I lost touch. I went into business, and Curlie went to university. Two years later he had a serious accident on a motorbike and ended up in Stoke Mandeville Hospital, seriously paralysed. I visited him in hospital once and was so shocked to see his wasted body and his bitter reaction to my visit. I have not seen or heard of Alan since, but I often think of him and hope that he was able to come to terms with his tragic experience and disability.

Finally, Chris Gibson. Chris was also in the rowing club and, somehow, in the fours and eights I was always rowing to the bow of Chris (rowing behind him) and my enduring memory of those days was the only sight I had: his badly shaped bottom on the sliding seat in front of me! Despite the fact that we also had little in common by way of interests other than drinking ale, Chris and I hit it off and spent many enjoyable times together. Chris was blessed with that quick Liverpool repartee, and I always remember the time we met for a pint after work in a pub in Upper Parliament Street, which is well-known to those who have frequented Liverpool. The pub was one of many in that area that were also B&B accommodation for commercial travellers. While drinking we chatted to a guy who was in Liverpool for the first time and he said:

> 'If you don't mind me saying so, my first impression of Liverpool is that it is the arsehole of England'.

Chris was a true Scouser and did not, as some may think, thump him one but responded:

> 'Just passing through, are you?'.

The joke seemed to pass over the guy's head, and I am convinced that he did not twig what Chris had said.

Chris met and married a lovely lady called Jacky who was a qualified barrister. I was privileged to be Chris's best man at their wedding and have stayed in touch on and off ever since. Chris and Jacky have two boys, Dan and Drew. Drew, who is the elder, at one point in his life had 'crashed out of uni', much to his father's disgust, and Alli and I took him under our wings. Drew is now a surrogate son of mine whom I love as much as my own. Very sadly, Jackie contracted breast cancer in her early forties and after a six-year fight died when Drew was sixteen and Dan his younger brother only eleven. We were all devastated. Chris has now remarried and lives in Northern Cyprus, so contact with him is very spasmodic.

As I recall those days, the striking thing is that each of my close friends and I had little in common, except friendship for each other. Maybe there is some Freudian or other psychological meaning whereby, like magnetism in Physics, like people repel while opposites attract!

So now it was the summer of 1962 and the A Level results were out. I had passed Biology, Chemistry, Physics and Art but, alas, my grades were not high enough to secure a place at medical school. I was offered places to take Biochemistry, Pharmacy or any of the pure biological subjects. I went for interviews at Evans Medical in Speke and GKN in Pinner, looking at the possibility of doing a sponsored sandwich course. But none of these options appealed me. My ambition of ten years had been dashed by a piece of paper from the examining board.

Over the next few weeks I must have been unbearable to my poor parents, who tried to encourage me; I moped around and, like most at that age, lay in bed until noon every day. After a few weeks of this, my father said to me that he had been speaking to a business friend of his who had his own marine insurance underwriting agency and was looking for a bright A Level school leaver to train in marine insurance. I remember telling my father (in a rather impolite and rude manner, as only a teenager would) exactly what I thought of his idea and where he could stick insurance. In 2010, some 50 years later, as a major shareholder and chairman of a very successful marine underwriting agency, I can just see my dear old dad up there looking down at me with a 'told you so' expression on his face. I recall that Mark Twain once said:

> When I was a boy of fourteen, my father was so ignorant I could hardly stand to have the old man around. But when I got to be twenty-one, I was astonished at how much he had learned.

My own father, understandably in a bit of a rage, said to me:

> 'Well you had bloody well better make your mind up and get yourself a job because you aren't going to spend the rest of your life idling in bed until noon every day'.

It was the first time in my life that I was faced with the question WHAT WOULD YOU LIKE TO DO? and I did not know the answer.

# Chapter 4
# WHO AM I?

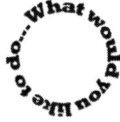

In the Army, all officers are subject to an annual Confidential report and at the end of this the commanding officer adds his comments, which are frequently short and to the point. At the end of the Confidential of one poor junior subaltern, who obviously was struggling to impress, his CO wrote:

> I would not recommend breeding from this officer.

That says it all!

Our character develops and our behaviour changes to a greater or lesser degree over the years under the influences of our environment and the people we meet. However, such development and changes in us do not affect what we are genetically. External influences, whether environment or the way that other people behave or treat you, cannot give you a talent that you have not genetically inherited. For example, if you have no tone or musical sense, no amount of teaching can make you into a Mozart. Similarly, this is true for people who are, or like me are not, naturally athletic. However, if you are fortunate enough to have inherited a real talent, then teaching and practice can help you hone it to perfection.

Despite recent advances in the understanding of genomes, the inheritance of genes and characteristics from generation to generation is still somewhat of a mystery. As I understand it, everyone inherits half their genes from each of his/her parents, so there cannot be an imbalance in percentage terms between father's and mother's genes which form the embryo and the eventual living person. It also seems true that each of us has more of a tendency to one 'side' of the family than the other. An example of this in my own family is that my sister is much more like our father in looks and character, whereas I take after my mother's side of our family. My mother told me that when I was a teenager she once glanced at me in half-profile. She was convinced that she was looking at her brother, my Uncle Leonard, as a teenager. I have experienced the same with my own children, in particular my son Duncan, who at times both in looks and behaviour was so like my wife's younger brother Donald (his uncle). Despite this, there are also some uncanny likenesses between Duncan and me, as you will see in some of my photographs. I am sure every reader will recall such experiences and understand my views about inheriting genes and their influence on the basic character of each and every one of us.

My father was a gentle, considerate man who passionately disliked anyone, especially in business, who was devious or dishonest. In this respect I am like him, but in other ways I believe that I have traits which I could not have inherited from him. Although he was a good middle manager, he lacked that ruthless ability that is essential for anyone in the higher echelons of business, and he would have been very uncomfortable in a more cut-throat environment. Maybe I am doing him an injustice, and if he had been more exposed to such he might have been different. It seems that he lived in an age when people were much more subservient to their superiors. This has never worried me, and I seem to revel in being a bit of a maverick in the face of a challenge, to the extent that there have been many occasions when I have gone out on a limb to try and enforce on others (often my superiors) what I considered to be the right thing to do. It was not for selfish or self-gain motives, and I was prepared to accept the personal consequences, however painful they might be. This sort of behaviour held me back in my career, since some of my superiors seemed to disapprove strongly of this behaviour. As an illustration, at MTS it was the tradition that the head boy put forward names recommended for vacancies as monitors at the end of each school term. I learned after leaving school that two head boys had put my name forward five times but I had been rejected by the staff committee because of my tendency to challenge rather than 'kow-tow' to authority.

I can only conclude that some genes are more dominant in the make-up of each of us. I do not mean those genes which are known to be dominant and determine such things as the colour of eyes or hair or skin pigmentation, but those which in certain combinations of your father's and mother's sides seem to predominate over the others to form your basic character.

In my case, I am convinced that a lot of my talents and faults come from my mother's side of the family, and I have searched to try and find an answer as to where they came from.

In the second chapter I mentioned Oliver Day, my grandfather's uncle who brought him up when my grandfather lost his parents. It is my Great Great Uncle Oliver who may have had an influence on my genetic make-up and my character. I could of course be completely wrong, but it's a nice idea!

My research into Oliver Day is limited. He was apparently a non-smoker and teetotal, so that rules out two similarities! As an entrepreneurial mill owner in Dewsbury, Yorkshire, he had a small milling business which was known locally as The Teddy Bear Factory. He made his money buying and importing the best astrakhan wool and weaving it into a material which he sold to the German teddy bear manufacturers Stieff. He was also a motor car fanatic, and made muffs for the ladies to wear while travelling in a motor car, also from astrakhan. He retired in 1930 having made a substantial fortune, and spent the last ten years buying and selling stocks and shares over his 'candle-stick' telephone. When he died he left a complex will. I was particularly amused by the penultimate clause in his will which states:

> I DIRECT that my Trustees shall after my apparent death and before my burial cause my body to be examined by some medical practitioner for the purpose of ascertaining whether or not I am really dead and that such medical practitioner shall sever such artery or arteries or perform such other operation as he may think necessary in order to ascertain that I am really dead.

Clearly Uncle Ollie did not have a great deal of faith in the medical profession. He was relying on the fact that his will would be read fairly promptly after his 'apparent death'. I am pleased to say that I have more faith in the doctors who will agree that I am dead, and less faith in solicitors that my will will be read so promptly.

In his will his nieces and nephews were the main beneficiaries, as well as loyal employees. My grandfather and his brother were the only beneficiaries to receive absolute inheritances; all the others were life-time beneficiaries. It was fascinating when, in 2008, I was contacted by Barclays Bank Trustees, following the death of a distant relative who was a spinster and had no direct descendants, to learn that her life interest was returned to the Oliver Day Trust to be distributed, and my sister and I, as the only surviving ultimate beneficiaries of our grandfather's will, received a small capital distribution from the Oliver Day Trust, some 60 years after his death. I wonder how long the Oliver Day Trust will run until all his legacies have been distributed.

Now I would like to set out what I believe are my main characteristics as a person. I believe that my positive traits are honesty, a positive attitude to life, loyalty and generosity. My bad points include that I am personally disorganised, have a tendency to leave things to the last minute, am intolerant of others and, especially, challenge those in authority, and I lack attention to detail. I am also a flamboyant and fun-loving person.

However, I do not wish to misrepresent or embellish myself, so I sought the opinion of Peter Nicholson Smith (PNS). PNS was my boss for over 25 years and perhaps the person who should best understand my character. This is how he sums me up.

When Peter approached me, he kindly sent me his ideas of his virtues, faults and likely behaviour in order to steer me in the right direction. Among these he picks out his liking for 'challenges—particularly to those in authority'. I think this request of me falls in this category. As usual there is the underlying assumption that **other** people will join in his 'current project' with zest and enthusiasm. Most of the time it has worked wonderfully, and Peter carried with him his ranks of the willing in his schemes—particularly where it contained an element of 'creating the big society' around the company and inside the company.

Peter joined Triumph Investment Trust Limited in the City from some job in Liverpool shortly before me at the end of 1968. I joined on April Fool's day the next year. In July 1979 I was appointed Managing Director and my life 'with Peter' really began. Managing directors like to be associated with 'doing things' and need people around them who get things started. Peter loved projects. He really had the drive to get things under way and to galvanise his team into action.

It was clear from the start that Peter had a tremendous flair for making firm friendships with directors and staff of the broking firms which we did business with. He loved and still does love entertaining—whether he can afford it or not—and his parties are always successful. I suspect Peter and I, in the background, might have been tougher on the underwriting front, but the operation was liked and respected locally. Peter always behaved uprightly and it worked.

Of course it didn't always work out as expected. I recruited Peter to run my 'management weekends'. As usual they were very successful most of the time. Peter's idea to give the attendees a nickname misfired as some considered them disrespectful. The Outstanding AEGON Delegate of the Year—the 'TOADY Award' which was a framed picture of me with 'you're wonderful' on it—went down like a lead balloon when it was presented to a Dutch colleague on our board who was 'insulted'. But they were fun ideas and most of the time the weekends really dealt with the day-to-day challenges we faced in the over-competitive insurance markets of the 1980s.

Peter was always straight and loyal, not only to his team but also to me. He was there when needed and never had to be told to work hard and the importance of reputation and selling ability to building up a new business. It was very reassuring.

I gave him the job of placing his own reinsurance of the Regional Office business and in particular the quota share reinsurance so vital to expanding underwriting capacity in the early days of any underwriting operation. He immediately recruited a very distinguished lady broker whose lovely employer had been 'ripped off' and together they made a spectacular job of a task of which Peter had no previous experience. His friends, of whom there seemed so many, rallied round. His reputation for telling it as it really was meant there were no unpleasant repercussions when results didn't always come up to scratch. No one deserted Peter's teams—the branch managers and underwriters and his reinsurers.

Of course Peter had his disasters directly as a result of his over-confidence and could get really low as a result.

Peter generally drove himself until he dropped in support of his family.

In thanking PNS for his contribution, I recall a quotation from the German 19th-century novelist John Paul Richter, who said:

A man never discloses his own character so clearly as when he describes another's.

*Touché*, PNS!

# Chapter 5
# INTO THE BIG BAD WORLD

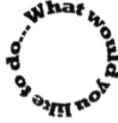

Thomas Edison once said:

I never did a day's work in my life, it was all fun.

The truth was that I did not know what I wanted to do! I was 18 years old and I thought I was grown-up, wise to life, determined to make my own decisions about my future, and that I could cope with the predicament that I now found myself in, having not got a place at medical college.

My logic was so flawed that, having said what I did to my father about insurance and working in an office, I replied to an advertisement in the *Liverpool Daily Post* for a junior trainee for Martins Bank Limited. I went for an interview and after this I was asked to take a handwriting test. I thought that having written my letter of application in longhand and with eight O Levels and four A Levels it was plainly obvious to anyone that I was capable of writing! I was to discover that a legible hand was an essential skill for working in the bank in those days, so that our customers could read and understand their hand-written statements. As I was also to find out, adding machines were also in short supply and mechanisation non-existent in the bank. Why I was not also asked to add up a column of figures I have never understood, but maybe the fact that I had O Level Maths was enough. I was offered a position as the 'junior' at Maghull branch at a salary of £230 per annum.

Maghull is a small town between Liverpool and Ormskirk, only eight miles from my parents' house and on a bus route. Having been a 'senior' person in a school of over 400 pupils and staff, I entered an office of five other people where I was not only the 'dog's body' but treated as such. This was a real culture shock. For the first four weeks all I was trusted to do was to file vouchers, make the tea and coffee, and go to the post office. It did not help that the guy before me had been an absolute disaster and had not filed any vouchers for weeks, so they were expecting me, even as an A Level school leaver, to be equally useless. I set out to prove them wrong and quickly gained their respect and was soon given other more responsible tasks such as handwriting statements and adding up the journal sheets (in £. s .d.). As a result I spent only six months at Maghull and was transferred to Blundellsands branch as a 'not quite so junior' member of the team of nine staff.

Blundellsands had some large commercial customers, as well as some very rich personal ones who had multitudes of dividends coming in for payment. The accounting was also 'mechanised'. The branch had Burroughs Sensimatic posting machines with magnetic stripes, which were about the nearest you could get to computers in those days. I quickly learned how to use the machines and was soon posting the entries to our customers' accounts and producing balances for the more senior staff to reconcile and agree.

Today, much is said about bankers' salaries and bonus payments. In those days all salaries were paid in the branch and not computerised, so I was able to see how much everyone else earned. There were large salary differentials in those days and even in a small branch of only six people my manager was paid a salary that was ten times that which I earned. You may not see the significance of this, but comparing it to today's standards I calculate that if a new 18-year-old employee started today on a salary of, say, £20,000, his boss (in an office of fewer than ten people) should be earning in excess of £200,000. This sort of differential no longer exists. What has happened is not that the boss is any worse off in real terms, but the rate of pay given to a junior or trainee employee is relatively much higher today and young people now have much more disposable income and buying power. From my first salary I drew out £5 each week in ten ten-shilling notes (ten shillings is equivalent to 50 pence) and gave my mother £2 10s, and the other half paid for my bus fares, cigarettes and a few pints of beer at the week-end with my friends, not much else.

Those of you who have a sharp brain will have realised that my weekly drawings were more than my income—£5 per week multiplied by 52 weeks was less than my £230 annual salary. At the same time that I started work I also joined Waterloo Rugby Club and signed on as an officer cadet in the TA, which not only gave me great fun but also paid me for training, so I was able to supplement my income to support my, not very extravagant, life style. My father, apart from disliking Service life, had a conscience about his time as a corporal armourer in the RAF during the war. He had loaded bombs on to aircraft which he knew would kill German civilians and could not understand that I wanted to indulge myself in the military life. I told Mr (Dai) Morgan, who was our school rugby master and CO of the CCF, that I wanted to join the TA. He, being an infantryman, said that he would arrange for me to have an interview with 5th Kings, the local Infantry TA Regiment. I told him that I would be more interested in being a tank than an infantry soldier. He kindly arranged for me to meet Colonel Mike Jeffries, who had just taken over command of 40/41st Royal Tank Regiment (40/41 RTR). Colonel Mike was a Regular professional soldier who had won his commission during the war and had a great influence on my early adult development. 40/41 RTR has not been in existence since the late 1960s, thanks to Harold Wilson (Labour Prime Minister in the 1960s) axing the regiment along with other TA units as part of a cost-saving budget. However, even now, some 40 years later, we still have a biennial reunion dinner and Col Mike is still going strong aged 89. Being an officer cadet was not easy, as I messed with the officers, where I was treated very much as the lowest of the low. At the same time I trained with the soldiers, who knew that I was seeking a commission and took every opportunity to give me as rough a time as possible. But again, it was all great fun and extremely good for character building.

Joining Waterloo Rugby Club was a real eye-opener. There is a big difference between school and club rugby. Waterloo in those days was one of the top clubs and ran a Schools XV in which people like me started and then either were pushed up into the 1st and 2nd XVs or dropped down into the other teams. This team was always captained by a past international player, and I was lucky enough to be tutored by Ned Ashcroft, who had been an English international back row forward in the early 1950s. Being a schoolmaster, Ned taught us the niceties of club rugby, rather than gamesman-like school rugby, and how to retaliate when necessary without incurring the wrath of the referee. I played for the 1st XV only once, when there had been a lot of injuries and an important county match coincided. Apart from that, mainly because I did not turn up regularly to training sessions, I languished in the lower echelons of the club and thoroughly enjoyed playing rough rugby.

As mentioned, I spent the first year in the TA as an officer cadet, during which time I was under scrutiny. I was in C Squadron, based in Bootle, and the OC was Major Tony Briscombe. Tony had undertaken National Service in Col Mike Jeffries' regiment and was not only a good OC but also a born leader of men, and was extremely well-liked and respected by all those both below and above him. Col Mike was often very critical that I was a little too 'gauche'. This made me try even harder. In May 1963, having been in for six months, we went to Tilshead on Salisbury Plain for our annual camp. This camp was put by Col Mike to training and I was on the troop commander's course, in charge of a troop of three tanks as part of squadron exercises. I took to this and really enjoyed the responsibilities and challenges which were presented. During one of the exercises, Tony Briscombe turned up at my tank in his Land Rover, jumped on the engine decks at the back of the turret and asked for my radio microphone. I duly passed it to him and to my amazement he transmitted:

> Charlie Charlie 3 Sunray has been taken out and call sign
> 31 is taking over command OUT,

and then handed the microphone back to me and said 'Get on with it, Peter'. He had just put me in charge of the squadron! Not thinking, I
immediately picked up the microphone and transmitted:

> Charlie Charlie 3 this is 31 SITREP over,

which meant that I was asking all the other 15 call signs now under my command to give me a 'situation report'. I did this just to give myself time to think, and by the time each of the other tanks and support sections had reported back to me where they were and what they were doing I had been able to compose myself and work out new instructions to control and continue the exercise. Apparently that turned out to be exactly the right action and Tony was very impressed at how I had handled the situation. At the end of camp, I was interviewed by a regimental selection board comprising the three squadron commanders and the adjutant, and was recommended for a commission, subject to a brigade interview board. At my end of camp interview with Col Mike, he said to me that if it had been his decision before camp he would not have recommended me for a commission, but he had been swayed by his squadron commanders and especially by the manner in which I had conducted myself on exercise. Wow! In September I attended the brigade board and in early October 1963 I was commissioned as Second Lieutenant P.B. Sangster on two-year probation and took command of my own troop of three tanks and 11 men.

As I have said, I loved the ceremonial occasions and, like most people, I particularly like military music. There were other benefits, and in particular the 1966 Football World Cup. One of the qualifying groups played at Goodison Park and the mass bands of the Liverpool TA regiments played before and during half-time. I happened to notice a circular asking for volunteers to be orderly officer on duty for each match, so I volunteered and was fortunate enough to be on duty for three of the matches, standing on the side-line and watching the boot of the great Eusebio help Portugal to progress to the knock-out rounds. Apart from when Liverpool played Everton away, these were the only occasions that I ever went to Goodison Park.

The next four years were real fun, and I progressed to second in command of Recce troop and then assistant adjutant and the less glamorous job of officers' mess secretary. In 1967, when Harold Wilson axed the TA, the regiment was merged with the Duke of Lancaster's Own Yeomanry in a civil defence role. Soon afterwards I married Alli and then moved to London, where I transferred to the Royal Armoured Corps pool of officers. In those days regular armoured regiments could not justify their war-time establishment, which required a second 'battle' captain in each squadron, and the pool provided this part-time establishment. As I was now a captain I was attached to 2nd Royal Tank Regiment. For the next 12 years we went to Germany every year to train for three weeks with 2 RTR on exercise, and once Alli, Penny (then five) and Duncan (aged three) all came with me to Munster in the middle of summer and attended the regimental ball. These were very happy times, but by the early 1980s my work commitment was making it increasingly difficult to continue and I resigned my commission, having had the Territorial Decoration conferred on me.

After 18 months at Blundellsands branch of Martins Bank, I was progressing well with my professional banking examinations and was transferred to Southport branch as a cashier. Southport branch was much bigger and busier than either of the two previous branches I had worked in, and had six young ladies of similar age to me who loved partying, so life was looking up. Within a further six months I had passed all my exams and was a qualified Associate of the Chartered Institute of Bankers. In those days this was no mean feat, as many of my work colleagues over the age of 30 were still struggling to complete their exams. I was to learn that this had not gone unnoticed in the personnel department. I was given the opportunity to train in security work, dealing with charges over assets to secure overdraft facilities at Southport, and looking after private customers' investment and stock market dealings. Southport branch had a sub-branch in the outskirts of the town, and when one day the clerk-in-charge was on holiday, Ike Clarke (himself a former war-time major who had been awarded the Military Cross) asked me to run the sub-branch for a week. Needless to say, I was flattered at such an expression of trust in my abilities, and jumped at the opportunity to take on such responsibility. I was only 22 years old.

During that week a customer of Liverpool City Office who was unknown to me came into the sub-branch to cash a cheque. That customer turned out to be Ian Buchanan, who was an ex-commanding officer of Liverpool Scottish Regiment (and a close friend of Col Mike Jeffries, my CO) and also the district general manager and local director of the bank—a very senior position. I must have impressed Ian Buchanan, because within six weeks I was transferred to Liverpool City Office as personal assistant to the bank's most senior manager. I was to learn that the bank had two fast-track posts for up-and-coming young employees. Personal assistant to the chief general manager always went to a graduate and my post to a non-graduate. I was given a salary rise well above normal. My job required me to sit in the same office as my new boss, Alec Tunnington. Alec was less than two years from retirement, and I was also to see the transition of his successor. I was required to learn shorthand (which I did) and sit in and take notes of meetings with the bank's top commercial clients, which included Royal Insurance, Cunard and other big shipping lines, and Mersey Docks & Harbour Board, and to construct minutes and then dictate them to a typist for recording. Alec Tunnington was also a JP and a trustee of numerous charities, and I was expected to maintain the books and accounts of the charities of which he was the treasurer, as well as look after his very busy diary. All this often involved long working days, but I relished the job and for the first time was exposed to and excited by the way big business worked.

I also decided that I would like to take accountancy qualifications to further my career prospects. The Chartered Institute was out of the question, as I would have had to leave the bank and take up articles. The Association of Certified Accountants, after great deliberation, decided that my work in the bank was 'not of an approved accounting nature' and refused me student membership.

While all this was going on in my business career, my mother had a good friend called Letty Rowe who lived only two roads from us. Letty had a daughter, Alli, who was the same age as me. Alli and I were frequently (but very much separately) invited to 21st and other parties or dances. Having met Alli on occasions, I had already decided that she was not my type, so imagine when my mother informed me that she had arranged with Letty that I would collect Alli and take her to a mutual friend's party so that Alli did not have to drive. And then proceeded to make the same arrangement with Letty several times again. Thanks, Mum! I did my duty politely, picking up Alli. She obviously reciprocated my feelings; the first time in the car she said that she did not expect that we would spend any time together at the party, which suited me, and we hardly spoke in the car. I spent my time at the bar with my mates, while Alli mixed with her friends, and then at the end I drove home and unceremoniously dumped her at her front gate. Alli, who had trained as a Cordon Bleu chef and a florist at Constance Spry's Winkfield College, had her own business, arranging flowers in the morning for a chain of up-market hotels and restaurants in the Liverpool and Cheshire area and, with two other girls, outside catering for dinner parties, hunt balls and other such up-market functions (not the sort of company I associated with).

After a couple of years, my mother informed me that Alli had got in a mess with her accounts and the tax man and that Mother had volunteered me to go and sort it all out for Alli. Thanks, again, Mum! So, like the dutiful son that I was, I begrudgingly went to Alli's house one Friday evening to look at the records and accounts. On arriving I made it quite clear to Alli that I had arranged to meet my mates for a pint at the Blundellsands Hotel at 9.00 pm so could not spend too long; she seemed quite happy with this. I am not sure what happened during the next two hours, but at 8.55 pm Alli said that, since I had driven her to parties before, she would be happy to run me to the Blundellsands Hotel and back home afterwards. A bit taken aback, how could I refuse such a generous offer? Alli knew that I was in the TA (a tank man) and in the car she told me that the previous Saturday she had been to a ladies night mess dinner with a friend of mine who was a subaltern in Vth Kings (Infantry) and that she had made a projectile from two cigar cases filled with matches and heated over a candle and that it had hit the commanding officer on the head. At about just the same time as she was telling me this she was behind a rather slow old driver in an even older car and said: 'I wish this b****y old fart would get a move on', and immediately accelerated past him on a slightly blind bend where, luckily, no one was coming the other way. I saw Alli for the first time in a different light, and rather warmed to her. We had a fun evening with my mates and I am not sure exactly what happened, but from that moment I actually looked forward to doing Alli's accounts and we spent a lot of time snogging and going out together, without saying a word to either of our mothers. The first time our mothers knew anything was when I invited Alli to a regimental function and made it clear to my fellow young officers that Alli was not available for dating.

Alli had enjoyed riding from an early age, was an accomplished rider and frequently went hunting with her friend, Boo Phillips. She had a mare called Eep and, while I had on occasions in the past sat astride a pony, Alli set about teaching me to 'ride properly' by giving me lessons on Eep. Alli was a hard task-master, and I remember falling off frequently and dismounting on more than one occasion with extremely sore muscles and my knees worn to the extent that they were bleeding. As a man, I was determined not to give in or be seen as a softie, so I persevered. Actually, I soon learned that there is no experience quite like sitting astride such a wonderful and powerful animal as a horse and being able to control its strength, a feeling of being king of the world. I wished that I had started earlier, and relished every opportunity to go riding with Alli, and even hunting a couple of times.

In a very short time Alli and I decided that we would get engaged and plan our marriage as soon as possible since we did not want a long engagement. We were engaged in June 1967 and soon after bought our first house, a three-bedroom semi in Freshfield, near Formby, which was in a poor state of repair, and set about renovating and re-decorating it. I had managed to save up a deposit of £300 from my TA bounty and the bank gave us a £3000 mortgage. These were busy and happy days, but in December I suffered what I thought was flu, which persisted and was diagnosed as infective hepatitis. I have no idea how I contracted this, which I understand is transmitted only by body fluids, and the only explanation I can think of is that I had been infected by another player's blood injury when playing rugby. However, it incapacitated me for three months and I remember suffering pretty serious depressions in January 1968. Further tests found that I was also suffering from gallstones and had a high blood cholesterol level. Sadly, also in January 1968 Alli's father died, having suffered from heart disease for more than 20 years. I, not being too well a bunny, was unable to do very much in planning our wedding and had been put on an alcohol—and fat-free diet for six months. I was signed off in June, just before my stag party, so it did not take much for my mates to get me drunk!

Our wedding took place on 6th July 1968, a lovely sunny day. Alli had decided on Sefton Church and that the time would be 2.30 pm, not realising that in those days this was closing time and right next door to the church was a nice country pub. The ushers were not in the best state to receive our guests, but the service went without a hitch! We had a pony and trap to take us to a lovely reception in a marquee in Letty's garden, and left to honeymoon in Jersey. We had a very happy 36 years together, albeit, as with all relationships, some ups and downs; in my opinion, anyone who says that their marriage or relationship never had any problems either is a liar or must be a very boring person.

My old boss, Alec Tunnington, had now retired and Donald Brewis arrived as my new boss. Donald and I did not exactly hit it off. He was a bachelor and a bit of a 'mummy's boy'—not what I had expected. Soon afterwards I was struck with infective hepatitis and off work for three months. When I returned to work, Donald had taken a liking to another young man who had stood in for me during my illness. My next career move was being planned, and it looked as if I would be returning to branch banking which, after my exposure to business at the top level, I did not relish. I was also told in confidence that Martins Bank and Barclays Bank were in merger talks, and I spent a few months acting as a courier, taking confidential documents by train from Liverpool to Barclays' head office in Lombard Street, London. The top management in Martins were selling this as a merger, but I could see that it was in fact a takeover by Barclays and would lead to fewer career opportunities, and it was likely that the Barclays men would get first consideration for prime jobs.

So there I was in the autumn of 1968, only two months married with a mortgage for the first time in my life, facing a move to a job which I did not want and felt would not better my career, working for a bank that offered fewer career opportunities than had previously existed and not being able to pursue further qualifications in accountancy. I was faced with that inevitable question: WHAT WOULD YOU LIKE TO DO?

I always read the *Financial Times* and one day in October I noticed a job advertisement for an assistant to the chief accountant of an acquisitive financial and banking group in the City of London.

I applied, went for interview and to my amazement I was offered the job. For the second time in my life I was faced with a major change of direction.

Apart from leaving the protective environment that I had had until then—living at home with Mum and Dad and working in an environment which I knew and was comfortable with—Alli, my wife of only four months, and I were faced with a period when I would be working away in London and returning home at week-ends, not knowing when or where we would move to in the alien South of England. My salary was to be trebled from £840 to £2500 per annum. This may seem a dream, but I realised that we would probably have to double both our mortgage and the interest rate (the bank had a low concessionary mortgage rate for staff) to buy a house in the south, and the cost of travel to and from work and the general cost of living would probably be higher.

This was the first, and as it turned out the only, time in my life that I was to write a letter of resignation from a job.

William James, an 18th-century American philosopher, once said about change:

> To change one's life:
> 1. Start immediately.
> 2. Do it flamboyantly.
> 3. No exceptions.

So I followed his advice.

# Chapter 6
# OF WOMEN AND WIVES

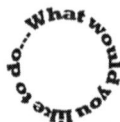

Some may have thought that so far I have made little mention of the ladies in my life, so I decided that I would devote a whole chapter to my two wonderful wives, Alli and Linda, and some of the women I have met, and the effect they have had on my life. Most of my experiences with the 'lassies' (to use one of Rabbie's immortal words) have been very happy; a few not quite so!

Soren Keirkegaard, a 19th-century Danish philosopher once said:

> To be a woman is something so strange, so confusing, and so complicated that only a woman could put up with it.

Throughout my life, a total mystery has been how the female brain works, and numerous discussions with my many men pals have confirmed that I am far from alone in this respect. After Alli died I decided to try and find an answer and, amongst other sources of potential explanation, I studied Bridget Jones in depth. All to no avail. To give some examples of the sort of things that have puzzled me:

Alli would say:

'Has someone forgotten to close a window?' when, in fact, what she meant was:

> 'It's a bit draughty; would you mind closing the window for me'!

Yet again, Linda one day was trying on a new dress that she had bought on one of her frequent shopping sprees. She stood halfway down the stairs and asked me my opinion. I said:

'That's fantastic darling, it makes you look so slim'.

Linda's response was:

> 'What, are you telling me that I am fat?'

You can't win!

It is also amazing that the whole female race seems to have a thing about lavatory seats being left up by men. Do they really get irritated about having to put it down when they want a wee, and have they never thought that men might find it irritating to have to lift the seat whenever **they** want a wee? Now I nearly always religiously put the seat and cover down when I have finished. I say 'nearly always' because sometimes I also deliberately do not rinse the washbasin after I have shaved. You have to let the ladies have some excuse to tell you off and nag, otherwise they get bored and start to lose interest. However, whenever Linda and I have a minor 'disagreement' (which I know I will not win) I always try to have the last word. This is usually:

'Of course, darling', or

'Whatever you say, darling', or even the more straightforward

'Yes, darling', or occasionally my reply is:

'But I am a man',

to which Linda will respond:

'That's no excuse',

and my retort is:

'I am not giving you an excuse, I am stating a fact'.

I am sure that I can be extremely frustrating and irritating, but it helps make life so much richer and more fun in the long run.

For my male readers who wish, I recommend that you occasionally quote to your wife Ephesians Chapter 5 Verses 22–24.

Ephesians Chapter 5. v22. Wives, submit to your husbands as to the Lord. v23. For the husband is the head of the wife as Christ is the head of the church, his body, of which he is the Saviour. v24. Now as the church submits to Christ, so also wives should submit to their husbands.

This is bound to wind her up, but I ask that you then read on and observe verses 25–2 and then both of you note verse 33.

Ephesians Chapter 5. v25. Husbands, love your wives, just as Christ loved the church and gave himself up for her v26 to make her holy, cleansing her by the washing with water through the word, v27 and to present her to himself as a radiant church, without stain or wrinkle or any other blemish, but holy and blameless. v28. In this same way, husbands ought to love their wives as their own bodies. He who loves his wife loves himself v29. After all, no one ever hated his own body, but he feeds and cares for it, just as Christ does the church.

Ephesians Chapter 5. v33. However, each one of you also must love his wife as he loves himself, and the wife must respect her husband.

I can honestly say that during my two marriages I never had any affairs. By modern standards you may think this a bit 'goody-goody' or even that there must be something wrong with me but, probably because of my upbringing and Christian morals, I have always believed in the sanctity of marriage. Yes, there have been times when I have flirted, and office parties (which I tried to avoid whenever I could) were always occasions when, with alcohol flowing, this sort of behaviour was almost expected and sometimes considered acceptable. Everyone enjoyed office gossip after such events, but I always made a positive effort not to let such flirting go any further than that.

So where do I start with my other women? The logical answer is my fantastic and loving Mum. She never forgave her parents for giving her only the one Christian name, Gladys, which she disliked intensely. After my father died she sold their house in Liverpool in which they had lived for over 20 years and moved to live in Somerset near my sister and her family, where she made new friends and was known to them as Jean.

Despite the feelings that both Brenda and I as children sometimes had, Mum always showed a fair, considerate and balanced attitude to us, and I really cannot remember any occasions when she overtly favoured either against the other on the many occasions that we had differences or squabbles. Mum was always fun-loving, and we used to say that after one gin and tonic she was anybody's, but after two gins and tonic she was nobody's! Mum had a great sense of humour that she had inherited from her father—my father, we always said, had a 'lavatory' humour. I think I was lucky enough to inherit these traits from both my parents. Mum also had some wonderful philosophical sayings and two which stick in my mind were:

> 'Make the most of life and enjoy it because it is not a dress rehearsal and you are a long time dead', and the other was:
> 'Aim for the stars and don't worry if you hit your head on the cowshed roof on the way up. It doesn't matter because at least you tried and you can pick yourself up and try again'.

Despite this, she was not at all happy when I left the bank and went to work in the City of London 'to seek my fortune in the streets paved with gold'. Her generation had survived the Depression of the 1920s and she was entrenched in the belief that a job with the bank was secure for life, with a good pension; how much changing times have proved her wrong. I think that she thought that I had moved into a more dodgy and dishonest business environment than working in the bank, because during her last few months, when she was a bit confused, she told me off for getting into 'bad company' and said she was very worried that I was doing some sort of 'shady business'. I found it very sad that she must have harboured this thought in the back of her mind for over 30 years but had never once mentioned it to me. More than anything, throughout my life the one thing that I never wanted to do was in any way let her down or do anything that either she or my father would be ashamed of. I loved Mum dearly and still do. She died in 2000 just short of her 92nd birthday.

My sister and I, as I mentioned in Chapter 2, had a bit of a love/hate relationship as kids (actually more a hate/hate relationship). Brenda went to an all-girls convent school and the one thing that we have always had in common was our Christian faith. This often did not show through in our behaviour when we were kids, but we found it easier to forgive and love each other as we grew up. Brenda was married to David when she was 18 and since then, apart from three years when we both lived in North Buckinghamshire in the late 60s/early 70s, we have lived miles apart and for many years saw each other only on occasional family get-togethers. To explain our relationship in early years, perhaps I can do no better than to quote an exchange of emails that I had recently with Brenda when discussing my book and our family tree. Brenda reminded me that she was born on Easter Sunday and that her birthday was the same day as that of our grandfather (Father's father who's name was Alex, hence Brenda's second name, Alexandra) and added:

'I was very special (until you came along!)'.

My reply to her, in jest, was:

'I am sorry that my 'coming along' ruined Easter Sundays. Not much I could do about that!'.

Brenda's reply was a bit unexpected, but I hope she will forgive me for quoting from it since it best summarises her side of the story.

'I was thoroughly spoiled in my first four and a half years of life living during the war in Southport with Mum, Granny and Granddad Ward and quite near to Granny and Granddad Sangster. Dad was away in the Air Force and only came home occasionally. So you can imagine my feelings when Mum had a darling son and you were then her pride and joy and everyone made such a fuss of you and seemed to forget me. I was so jealous of you, for which I am very sorry, but it was not my fault, just circumstances. As you grew a toddler and small boy I always had the job of looking after you and got into trouble every time you got hurt. It was always my fault, whether it was or not. I know I was sometimes quite hard on you, and for this I am very sorry, but because I was always blamed I developed a guilt complex and resented you all the more. However, having said all that, we had some good times together as we grew up and we were both very fortunate to have such good parents and grandparents who passed on many healthy genes and lots of good advice.'

My reply was:

'I was really joking in my comments about ruining your Easter Sundays! And you did not need to say some of those things. I know that you love me and I you dearly, although perhaps we have not shown it openly enough to each other! None of us are perfect—I was also a bit of a little brat most of the time'.

Over the past 20 years Brenda and I have made a special effort to meet much more frequently, and I am very happy that we are now very close to each other and have a lot of fun when we meet, especially with her lovely family.

So now onwards! as I am sure that you would like to read some more juicy bits about my relationship with ladies.

I have already referred to my late teens and early 20s when I was in a youth choir, which was formed by one of my best school friends, Gerry Brown, from some of us who were in St Michael's Church Choir, and others soon joined. We were a very professional four-part choir and used to compete with a good degree of success in music festivals in Lancashire and North Wales. We also enjoyed carol singing at Christmas and were regularly rewarded by invitations into people's houses in the Blundellsands ('posh') area and plied with mince pies and drinks. This was also the first time following puberty that I had been exposed at close quarters to the fairer sex. Anne, who was a student nurse at Moorfield's Eye Hospital, joined the choir and I took a bit of a fancy to her and tried to chat her up in the hope that we could form some sort of relationship. Maybe the fact that Anne was a nurse appealed to me (my male readers will probably understand this) and here I am some 40+ years later happily married to Linda, who was a nurse all her life and often wears theatre greens to go to bed in; aren't I a lucky man! Anne did not reciprocate my feelings, and after a lot of effort I had to retire rather hurt, but we still remained friends.

This episode left me somewhat disillusioned (whether it was from being rejected or that I had lost my confidence) and I decided that I would no longer try to make the running and vowed never to get serious again with anyone of the opposite sex. At about the same time I had left school, taken up playing rugby and joined the TA. This meant that Saturdays were lost with morning work and afternoon rugby followed by copious drinking, and Sundays with TA training. Maybe because of this and my change of attitude it seemed that I did not have to search, and opportunities presented themselves from girls seeking me out. I had a whole string of dates, and I prided myself on never taking the same girl twice to a regimental cocktail party, dinner or other parade or celebration where ladies were invited. My fellow officers soon cottoned on, and some of them brought my ex-dates to subsequent regimental functions and my OC in C Squadron nicknamed me the 'regimental pimp'. One of my colleagues dated Jane, one of my ex one-off dates, and they subsequently married and are still happily married with a grown-up family and grandchildren.

I have already explained how Alli and I met each other and fell in love and married. We were married on 6th July 1968 and, sadly, Alli died in November 2003 following a number of years suffering from heart disease. Her father and two of her brothers had also died at around the age of 60 from heart-related infirmities, so there was obviously a genetic connection with their early deaths. Our years together, with our two wonderful children growing up, were very happy, albeit with a few difficult times, and I mention most of these experiences in other chapters. I loved Alli dearly and still do, and I miss her and the fun and happiness which she gave me during our 36 years together.

My daughter, Penny, has given me many years of happiness, and at times immense frustration. Penny had a passion for animals, and especially horses, from an early age. When she was just two years old she awoke one evening at about 10.00 pm and we brought her into the lounge for a while because we were watching the Horse of the Year show on television. She sat glued to the screen as Harvey Smith was jumping, and as he crashed into a fence and was unceremoniously dumped on the ground by his mount, Penny, with a poker face, said:

'Dropped it'.

The other thing that sticks in my mind about Penny when she was a child is that whenever Alli or I asked Penny and Duncan who had done something Penny would always immediately respond with:

'It wasn't me'.

I would say:

'I didn't ask who it wasn't, I asked who it was'.

Typical woman: Penny would never admit to anything!

Her adult life has been dominated by her career with horses, training and eventing them. From the start she was determined to succeed, passing her Pony Club A Test with distinction and qualifying as a BHS AI before she was 21. Having trained in Ascot in a dressage yard, she then went to work for British International Event rider Karen Dixon (née Straker) as head girl. Penny is now a British Eventing Instructor and is looking to gain her full BHS instructor qualification. Eventing has taken its toll on Penny, with more broken bones than you can imagine, but this never stalled her determination to get back on the horse and get on with life as soon as possible. She still devotes long hours to caring for horses, training and competing, as well as teaching others horsemanship. This leaves her with little time for having what most people would call a 'normal' life, but she always rises to the occasion, she scrubs up well and is a very beautiful, fun-loving lady.

I was delighted when recently on her birthday her partner John proposed to her. I will enjoy giving my daughter away in June 2011, while I hope I will still have good health. However, I suspect that there will be no pitter-patter of tiny feet, just the continuing clip-clop of horses' hooves.

In business life I have met and been greatly influenced by many women at all levels, and in Chapter 9 I express my views about women in management. However, there are a few whom I would like to mention since they have affected me during my working career. I was brought up in the private secretary/typewriter/dictation era which, thanks to the computer and word processing, is now very much a thing of the past. In some ways this is a pity, as I was fortunate enough to experience three wonderful ladies who at one time or another were my secretaries. First, Freddie was my secretary when I was administration and personnel manager in the early

1980s. Freddie later went on to be personnel officer and was a very competent and loyal person. She would not just take things at face value, and always challenged me when she felt that things were not quite right. I remember that I had a yucca plant in my office which she took a dislike to. Despite this, it grew well and, now planted in the garden, is over 12 feet tall. Freddie and her husband, Trevor, are now retired and live in St Lucia. Freddie always did like the sunshine. When I was in charge of the Liverpool and later Manchester offices my secretary was Gill. Gill was without doubt the most efficient person I have known. Whenever I had a meeting, all the files and papers were on my desk in good time for preparation without my having to ask, and her ability to organise travel and accommodation was faultless. Finally, Doris was my secretary when I was a director of AEGON. Doris was older than Freddie and Gill with two grown-up children, having been widowed and then experienced an unhappy second marriage. Doris was a wonderful person who, because she spoke fluent Dutch, was a great asset in dealing with colleagues from our parent company. Doris now lives and works in the Netherlands.

Enid I recruited as reinsurance manager to take the load of placing our reinsurances off me. Enid was well-connected in the reinsurance industry and a very competent reinsurance professional, as well as being a very good manager. Enid is also now retired with her husband Jimmy, and I still keep in touch with them as good friends. I will also briefly mention Janet, who was chartered accountant and managing director of a service company that I had some dealings with when I was trying to seek new ventures during the later 1990s. In my view, a lot of chartered accountants seem to have an over-inflated opinion of their abilities to organise and manage people. In my usual flamboyant style I always entered their office saying 'Good morning, ladies' to the staff. For some reason, Janet took exception to this and in a rather blunt and unpleasant manner told me to desist from calling her female staff 'ladies'. This was one of the few times in my life when I was lost for words, although I felt like asking Janet 'If they are not ladies, what are they?'

I cannot complete this chapter without mentioning Linda. I often say that I am the luckiest man, having found and enjoyed the love and fellowship of two wonderful wives. Alli was a hard act for anyone to follow.

Andy Ripley, in his book *Ripley's World*, talks of the evening of 25th November 2005 when I and my fellow directors in Lead

Yacht had dinner at the Cavalry and Guards Club at 127 Piccadilly with our wives. This was soon after Andy had been diagnosed with prostate cancer, and he says:

> ". . . everybody has their own secrets, their own issues, their own concerns, their own stuff. For example, at the dinner at 127 Piccadilly . . . I discovered that Peter had met his new wife (both were recently bereaved) through an Internet site and had proposed to her within 13 days and that, against all expectations, he and Linda were really happy."

I would never describe Andy as one who makes understatements, but perhaps this was one. After finding each other through a matching web site and 'chatting' for some four weeks, Linda and I met in a café one Saturday morning and I experienced that 'chemistry' which I had not felt since the time that Alli drove me for a drink to the pub in 1966. And, yes, it is true that I proposed to Linda only 13 days later. I cannot find words to describe the joy and happiness that Linda has given me since we first met. I will mention all this in more detail in Chapter 12.

Andy then goes on to say:

> I really should take every opportunity to keep my mouth shut and listen. If people know she [in Andy's book he refers to his cancer as 'the other woman', or in this context 'she', who is trying to tempt him to 'come to him' and he is fighting her off!] is inside, you don't have to tell them, they know. Just do what women have been doing since time began: be a pair of ears and simply listen. That'll keep those invites flowing.

# Chapter 7
# BIG CHANGES

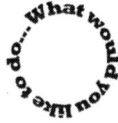

*What would you like to do...*

I had left the security of a job in the bank and ventured into the unknown territory of the big City of London. What on earth had I done? How were Alli and I going to cope?

I decided that the best advice from William James (see end of Chapter 5) was:

Do it flamboyantly,

and flamboyant is something that I have always found a natural thing to be.

My sister Brenda and her husband David lived just outside Bletchley in North Buckinghamshire (now part of Milton Keynes) and they very kindly agreed to lodge me from Monday to Friday until Alli and I sold our house and moved, as Northerners would say, 'down South'. I bought myself a Vespa scooter to get me the four miles from Brenda and David's house to Bletchley Station, and I used my riding bowler hat as protection on the motorbike. I turned up every day at the office in Copthall Court in the City in my bowler hat, pinstripe suit, starched collar and British Warm (officers' military) overcoat.

I had technically worked for Barclays Bank for two days, but on 3rd December 1968 I started as personal assistant to Uri Hyde. He was by birth a Hungarian Jew, whose family had fled to the UK before the war to escape the threat from Nazi Germany, and was the chief accountant of Triumph Investment Trust Limited, a financial and banking group which *Private Eye* in one of its articles referred to as Nipple Limited (short for TIT Limited). I found myself in a completely strange environment, taking a job in which I had no real experience and in the City, a place that I had only previously read about in awe as **the** financial centre of the world. Flamboyancy was my best friend! One of the first things I did was to contact John Fleming, an old TA colleague who was also flamboyant and now lived and worked in London. The following week I met him after work in a pub in Shepherd Market. As I arrived there it was snowing heavily. This early memory of a romantic London I will never forget, and John's company and advice over a pint of beer gave me strength for the challenges ahead.

After Christmas, Alli joined me, staying with Brenda and David in North Bucks, and Alli and I set about house hunting. On New Year's Eve, Brenda persuaded Alli to come off the pill and the result was that Penny was born 11 months later. We found a house, which was a unit in a converted old coach house about two miles from Brenda and David. Alli's mum had decided to sell the old family house which, after Alli's father's death and our marriage, she felt was too large for her on her own. She bought our house in Formby from us and lived there until she died over 30 years later at the age of 93. In April 1969, with Alli now pregnant, we moved into our new house and were able for the first time to start building our marital home together.

Before we were married, Alli had given her horse, Eep, to a friend, and we bought a gentlemanly grey gelding called Charlesworth which Alli and I took turns to hack out. Charlesworth was wonderful, but refused totally to jump. Whenever Alli or I took him to a local show he let us down, often dumping me unceremoniously on to the ground at the first jump! Now with Alli's pregnancy and my having time only at week-ends, we decided to sell Charlesworth to a local riding school. We also had an MG Midget sports car for the summer of 1969, and I remember that Alli's somewhat rotund stomach from bearing Penny rubbed on the steering wheel when she drove it. Soon after Penny was born Alli and I were still hankering after horses, so we went to the New Forest and bought two ponies in the sales with the idea of breaking them so that Penny could learn to ride. Looking back, this was rather an ambitious and somewhat foolish project, bearing in mind my business pressures and with the prospect of a new baby, but you do silly things when you are young.

I had now been accepted as a member of the Association of Certified Accountants and started my correspondence course for the exams. I am sorry to say that, although I continued with my studies for the next two years, I then gave up. I got to my finals but failed the taxation exam. In those days there were four exam subjects at each stage, and if you failed one you had to re-sit all of them at the next sitting, six months later. I was then working long days, and had a young family and little time to study and see the family, and I decided not to continue with my accountancy qualifications. However, the exams I had passed were of great benefit to my further understanding of accountancy and company law which has ever since held me in good stead.

The first three months of 1969 were frantic for me at work. I was responsible for the consolidation of the group accounts, work which I had never done before but which I cottoned on to quickly. I had two bookkeepers working for me. Janet was about my age and a very competent lady; the other was Katie, who was elderly and a bit slow. Katie was from an East German Jewish family and had been in Auschwitz, where she lost both her parents. She rarely talked about her experiences other than to show us the number tattooed on her arm, but for the first time in my life I realised the horror of the Holocaust, and I hope that people will never forget how cruel humans can be to each other. I also went to Jersey for two weeks to learn about the workings of the off-shore bank owned by Triumph.

Then something happened on April Fool's Day 1969 which would turn out to have a profound effect on my business life and career.

Peter Nicholson Smith (ever to be known as PNS) arrived at Triumph as financial director and my new boss.

Little was I to know it, but as it happened I was to work for PNS for the next 25 years and he is still a real friend to this day. PNS's character will become obvious in the ensuing chapters but, to set the scene, he is a boisterous and loud person (he says this was only to overcome his underlying shyness, but I am sure that it is part of his inherited character) and has a brilliant brain—a First from Cambridge, a chartered accountant (in the top ten of his final examinations) and when, as he explained to me, during his intermediate year in articles as a trainee accountant:

> 'There was something missing in my life and when I analysed it I realised that for the first time in over 15 years I did not have any exams to sit. So I went back to Cambridge and saw my old tutor and in a week studied for and obtained an honours degree in International Law'.

Not long after PNS arrived, Triumph acquired an insurance company and PNS was appointed to the Board as the group director. That morning he summoned me to accompany him to meet the managing director, the previous major shareholder of the company, Ralph Delborgo. Ralph was a bit abrupt about the fact that PNS was an accountant and knew nothing about insurance. We came out of the meeting and PNS frog-marched me to the Chartered Insurance

Institute where he enrolled on the spot as a student. In less than a year he had qualified as a Fellow of the Institute despite the fact that he failed a law paper and, when he questioned this with the Institute in the light of the fact that he had a law degree, was given an exemption from the subject after 'failing'. At the next board meeting PNS said:

> 'Don't you ever dare say to me again that I know nothing about insurance'.

Over the next two years I was involved in pre-acquisition investigations and post-acquisition 'sorting out' of accounting systems of subsidiaries to bring them into line with group standards. PNS frequently tasked me to work at various newly acquired subsidiaries on a variety of other organisational and management improvement assignments. I was not always working on my own, and often under the guidance of more experienced colleagues, but the challenges this work presented and the excitement I got from it were truly stimulating.

While this was going on at work, on 10th December 1969, Alli gave birth to our daughter Penny. She was born with light-ginger hair. This was a bit of a shock to us as the milkman had ginger hair, but then we remembered that he was going out with the window cleaner! Only 14 months later our son Duncan was born. My lady readers will imagine what Alli must have gone through, and what a handful this must have been, especially with my working long hours and little able to help except at the week-ends. In sympathy for Alli, on the advice of Alli's eldest brother Mike who told me that I had a 'rich man's family'—one of each—I decided, much to the relief of Alli's mother who was already a grandmother of ten and worried about us continuing to 'sprog' every year or so, to have a vasectomy. This was a fairly new procedure at that time and a brave decision to make. Because we lived so far out of London, I was leaving home before 7.00 am in the morning, before Penny and Duncan were awake, and getting home after 8.00 pm at night when they were in bed asleep. So for the first six-odd years of their life I am sure that they must have thought that Daddy was that 'strange' man who came to stay with Mummy at the week-ends. During our married life I devoted all my spare time to spending it with Alli, Penny and Duncan and their interests, rather than pursuing any personal activities that I could have taken a fancy to. This is why, among other things, I never tried to take golf too seriously and only occasionally hacked around at business or other corporate arranged golf matches.

Alli and I had moved in 1971 from our house near Bletchley to a small thatched cottage in a village called Emberton near Olney. It was at the end of a lane and was an idyllic home. We spent four very happy years and made numerous friends whom I still keep in touch with, albeit frequently only by exchanging news in Christmas cards. We were very much involved in village life and with friends raising money for the local school and other charities. On one such occasion, at Alli's mum's suggestion, we organised a 'live' Punch and Judy Show one evening in aid of the village school. We constructed a large Punch and Judy stall and I was Judy (made up from the waist upwards) and other parents took on the other roles. The script was written in rhyming doggerel by Mike Watts, a local solicitor. I recall that the opening lines, which Mike had as the deckchair man, suitably dressed in an old fashioned bathing costume, were:

'Hello boys and girls, you know who I am',
to which we all chorused:

'Yes, you're the Punch and Judy Man'.

The rhyming got worse and all the characters were skits on local personalities. One of the 'actors' was John Hague who is quite tall and was the policeman called 'Watt's the Law'. It was all great fun. John Hague, his wife Judy and their son and daughter still keep in touch and we still get together on occasions despite their living in North Yorkshire.

It was at Emberton that Penny started school and Duncan first went to nursery classes. On Duncan's first day Alli received a phone call asking her to collect him, as he had been a disruptive influence. When Alli asked what Duncan had done wrong, she was told that he had taken a liking to a little blond girl and would not stop kissing her under the desk.

'Good lad—a chip off the old block', was my reaction. However, he was allowed to return the next day. I do not know whether he no longer fancied the girl or just behaved a bit better, but there were no more problems. One Sunday in the summer Alli and I held a lunchtime party in our garden. When most of the guests were leaving at about 4.00 pm I returned to the garden to encounter a rather giggly and staggering son. Duncan had gone round finishing off all the dregs in the glasses left by people. I can vouch for the fact that he hasn't changed! Penny was already showing signs of wanting to learn at school, and of the love of animals, particularly horses. We had the two New Forest ponies, which we had bought as yearlings at the sales. Penny loved riding (then on a leading rein). One of our neighbours kept goats and we all fell in love with these animals, so we started keeping two goats as companions for the ponies, and they provided our milk supply. These were happy years, during which we saw Penny and Duncan grow from being babies to becoming their own characters. Alli's mum and my parents visited us. I remember we were sitting after Sunday lunch on a sunny day once and the kids (aged three and two) had left the table and were playing around the house. My mother looked out of the dining room window and said 'It's raining'. I burst out into laughter immediately, realising that Duncan was piddling out of one of the upstairs windows.

In 1973, I had started an investigation exercise at what was now Triumph Insurance Company, the newly acquired subsidiary of the Triumph Group. The idea was to identify unclosed business which had been written over the past ten years. I was amazed at how inefficient and slip-shod the London insurance market was in its administration and accounting practices at the time. Underwriters would quote or even write business through brokers and there would be no follow-up to ensure that the business was actually closed and premiums paid, or whether an outstanding quote had been taken up or not. My task was to set up an investigation and try and find premium income which had not been closed. I designed a set of manual procedures to carry out this task and employed on a temporary basis 12 ladies who had previously given up work to start a family but then wanted part-time work while their children were at school. The task lasted nine months and had varying success, but by that time our managing director was so concerned about general procedures in the company that, at the beginning of 1974, he asked me to transfer from the Group to a permanent appointment as organisation and methods manager for the insurance company and to take over control of the computer processing which was contracted to a bureau. My boss, PNS, who was also a director of the insurance company, agreed to my appointment.

1975 was a year which many either have not experienced or may not recall. You may think that the economy and possible recession of 2010 following the world banking crisis were worrying, but in 1974/1975 the world was also in serious financial recession. Inflation in the UK was 24.2% (in 1974 inflation had already reached 17.2%

and our company had given staff three pay rises just to keep up). There was an oil crisis with a severe shortage of fuel and the threat of rationing and rocketing prices; the cost of petrol more than doubled in price. The FTSE 100 index fell to 25% of its previous value in just three months following a fringe-banking crisis in the UK at the end of 1974 which had resulted in Triumph Investment Trust, the group for which I worked, going into liquidation. The IRA made several attacks on London, including bombing the Hilton Hotel. The *Sex Discrimination and Equal Pay Act* became statute and Margaret Thatcher became the first female leader of the Conservative Party. Also in that year Bill Gates and Paul Allen formed Microsoft and registered the name as a trademark, and Tiger Woods was born. On balance, 1975 will always stand out in my memory as probably the worst in my lifetime.

Luckily, the directors of Triumph Insurance, before the collapse of the Triumph Group, had ring-fenced the insurance company's assets for the benefit of the policyholders, and the liquidator of the group could not use these funds for the purpose of paying fees, Group creditors or shareholders. The only way that value could be realised from the insurance company subsidiary, therefore, was to sell it as a going concern, and the liquidator sold it to a Dutch insurance group called Ennia. All our jobs were secure and a new chapter started in our lives.

Ennia was a progressive and ambitious group and had acquired a subsidiary in the London insurance market, which was always, and still is, considered to be **the** insurance centre of the world and a prestigious place to be involved in. They were anxious to help us progress while, as is natural to the Dutch, saving on costs. We used to say:

> 'the trouble with working for the Dutch is they pay too little and expect too much'.

Things moved very fast, but not without full consultation and involvement of the management and staff, for the Dutch were streets ahead of the UK in employee consultation and involvement. Within nine months we had acquired a new administrative office building in Edenbridge in Kent to which 80% of the staff were offered relocation or the alternative of a generous redundancy package. The company purchased its own mainframe computer, taking in-house our data processing, which had previously been contracted out. I was later to learn that the capital investment for all this was £2 million, but the long-term annual savings were in excess of £1 million, so it was a very shrewd investment. I was appointed data processing manager, reporting to PNS, who had just been appointed a director and charged with the task of setting up the whole in-house computer operations.

Adam Wilson, who had been a consultant working for us, was appointed systems manager. From the first time I met Adam I had nothing but total respect for his superior intellect, and Adam has often said to me that he had total respect for my talent for making a decision, getting on with a task and making it work, rather than sitting back and analysing all the potential pitfalls before taking any action, as was his nature. This mutual understanding was the secret to our success, and because of our different strengths and weaknesses we made an excellent team. Adam and I went on to have many happy years working and bantering with each other. Although our paths have gone in different direction over the past 15 years and we have lost close touch, we still meet occasionally and enjoy each other's company. The taking in-house of our data processing involved both of us in long hours (once I left home for work and did not return until 36 hours later, having worked through the night) and, including a trial three-month parallel running, it took us less than four months to complete. This was a resounding success—a feat that would do nothing but good for Adam's and my long-term career prospects. We both, through different routes and with sometimes conflicting opinions and talents, went on to become fellow directors of the company.

Apart from Allan Norton (who features later in my story), Adam is the only person I have ever worked with where there has been such an absolute mutual respect for and trust in each other's abilities. We never challenged each other's decisions or recommendations, but on occasions would ask each other's views on issues about which either of us had some doubts. This is the mark of true respect and trust, which is a rare experience in life and something to be cherished.

Even more to be cherished was Allan, who trusted me to an extent that I felt on occasions anyone else would have considered too risky or even possibly foolish, and the faith he has shown in me (as I in him). I will never forget and will be forever grateful for Allan's love and friendship.

I also was to be relocated in my job, and Alli and I set about seeking a new house somewhere in Kent, Surrey or Sussex. The thatched cottage in North Bucks had two acres of land and outbuildings, and it soon became obvious that we could not afford to buy a house in the south-east with a decent amount of accommodation for a family and anything more than a reasonable garden plot. We therefore decided to sell the two ponies and found a small four-bedroom detached house with an outbuilding that could house the goats in a village called Tandridge near Oxted in Surrey, less than ten miles from the new office in Edenbridge and easily commutable to London. When we moved, the two goats travelled in the back of my VW estate car and their pee dribbled out of the back of the car as we drove through London on our journey (the M25 was then only part complete and useless for a circular journey around London). Tandridge village, like Emberton which we had just left, had a very strong community, focused on the church and the church-sponsored primary school. We settled in quickly to the village life, and Penny and Duncan loved their new school. For the first time in their lives (and mine) I was able to see them off to school and spend precious time with them after work and before bed-time.

To be able to have the time to react to and play with your children as they grow up is a precious gift to be relished and not one to be squandered; this experience is a one-off chance in life and if not taken can be lost for ever. Alli and I loved animals, and I cannot remember ever living in a house without at least one dog in it. We still had a hankering to be able to keep ponies for Penny and Duncan, but did not have the land, so soon after settling in we decided to buy four ducklings. This was the summer of 1976, which was one of the few heatwave summers. Alli said that ducks needed water. I got a big shallow bowl and filled it with water in the garden and put our newly acquired ducklings in it. We went shopping and returned an hour later to find all four ducklings floating dead in the water. How can you drown ducks? Penny was a bit upset, and so we went to see some sheep at the nearby farm and ended up buying two to fatten up on surplus goat's milk. After 18 months, we found a house with three and a half acres just outside East Grinstead and moved again and went back 'into horses'. This has lasted ever since and, although for a few years now I have not been involved with the day-to-day problems of the horse world, it was to become Penny's love and life, which I will say more about later.

Meanwhile, at work the move from London had been a success. I had recruited an organisation and methods analyst called Peter Woodhouse to work for me. Peter had served a short-service commission (three years) in the Royal Artillery before training as an O&M analyst. Peter was a good and hardworking chap. I felt that I had always been quite capable of bullshitting, but Peter was a past master and expert by comparison. As part of the company move to Edenbridge there was a need for a personnel manager. Peter was taking professional qualifications in personnel management and I was delighted when he was promoted to this position, because he was excellent at recruiting and training staff to replace those who had decided to accept redundancy rather than re-locate. This was no mean task, since more than 50 jobs (mainly junior or clerical positions) out of a total staff of 120 had to be recruited from a not very large local workforce. However, in 1979 Peter found a more senior job with better career prospects and resigned. I was asked by the directors if I would take over the job of personnel manager, coupled with the general administration of the Edenbridge office. This was not on my list of career moves, as I had set my sights on progression, ideally into underwriting, and moving upwards into a more responsible position rather than what I saw as a sideways move to a job which had been vacated by someone I had recruited and trained. I turned down the post.

PNS, who had just been appointed managing director of the company, took me to one side and had quiet words with me. He understood my frustrations. The company was experiencing high turnover of staff and low morale. This is not unusual where, having four years earlier recruited 50 new staff, a larger than normal proportion were 'job-hoppers' and the company was starting to suffer from this effect. PNS felt that I would be the ideal person to deal with these problems. He also told me that the company was planning to open regional offices and that the first would be in Liverpool, for which a new manager had been already been recruited. PNS was to have Board responsibility for this business development and I would be reporting to him. Part of my new job would be to find an office in Liverpool, recruit the staff and then be involved with opening and marketing other new offices in the UK over the next three years.

My parents were ageing now and still lived near Liverpool. My father, in particular, was suffering from emphysema, so this would give me an opportunity to stay with them on my visits and spend more time with them.

Again I was faced with that inevitable question:

## WHAT WOULD YOU LIKE TO DO?

With reluctance, and taking PNS at his word, I agreed. I cannot say that I particularly enjoyed my job during the next four years, except organising functions, entertaining brokers and developing new offices in the UK, but the experience gained in the many problems of personnel management and human resources stood me in good stead in the years to come.

Agnes De Mille, an American dancer surprisingly once said:

> No trumpets sound when the important decisions of our life are made. Destiny is made known silently.

It was to turn out that the trust I placed in PNS, and his continued support over the next ten years, were to pay off in my future career progression.

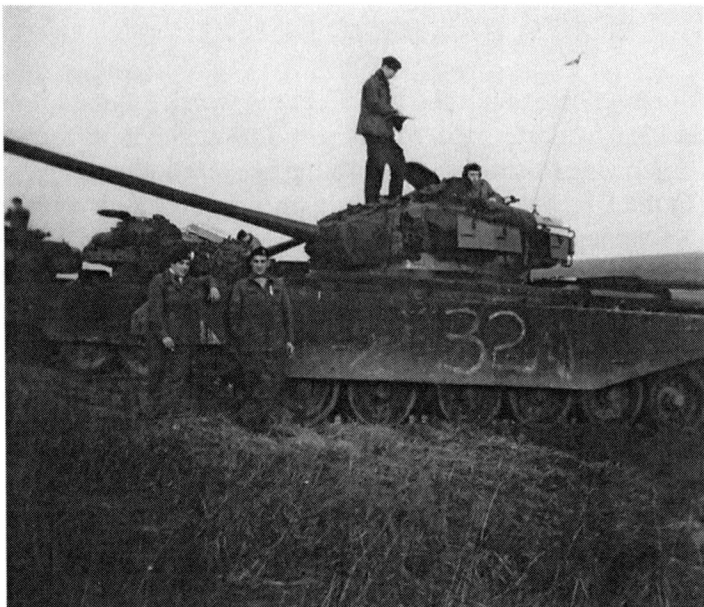

*Officer Cadet Peter Sangster on call-sign 32. 1963*

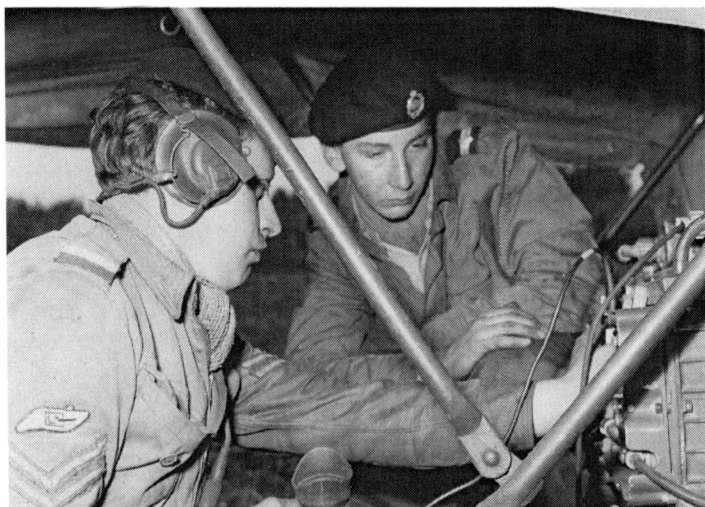

*2nd Lt Peter Sangster. 1964*

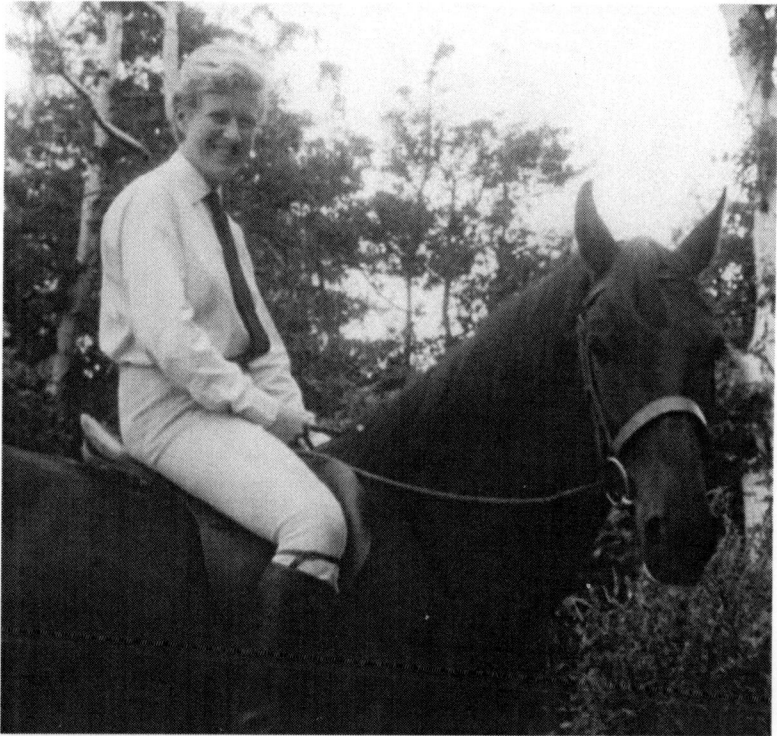

*Alli, before we were married on her horse "Eep". 1967*

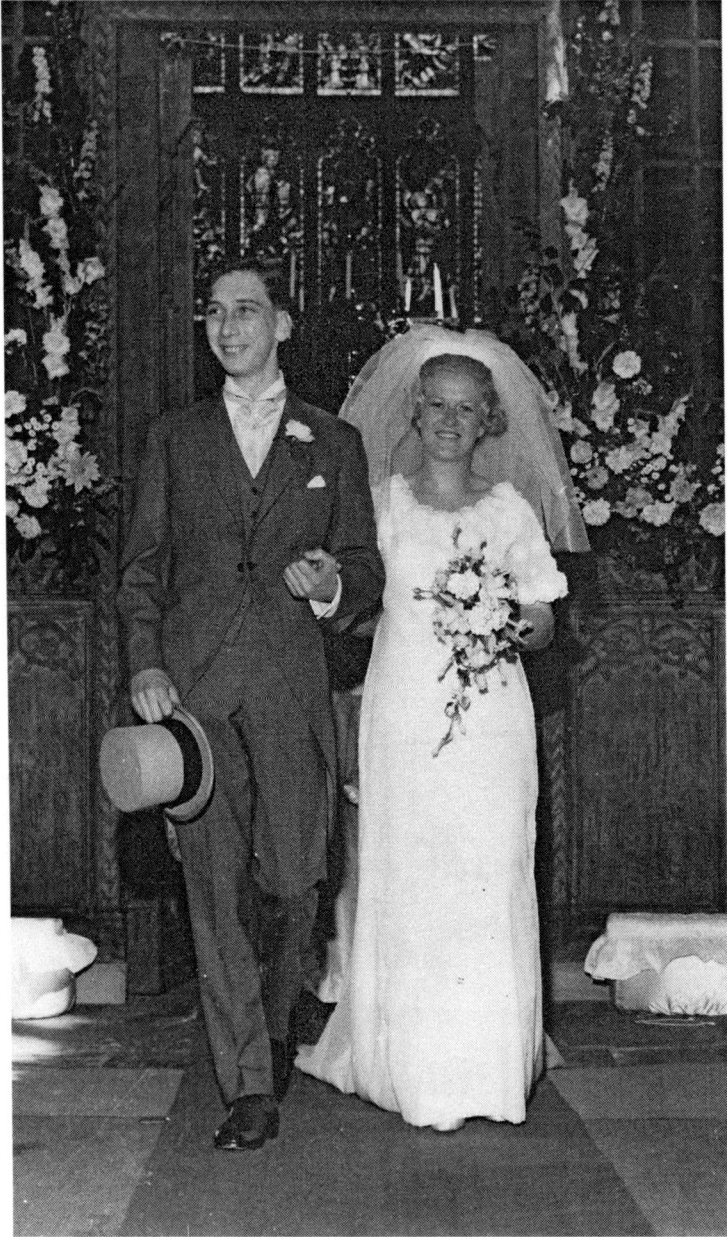

*Alli & Me 6th July 1968*

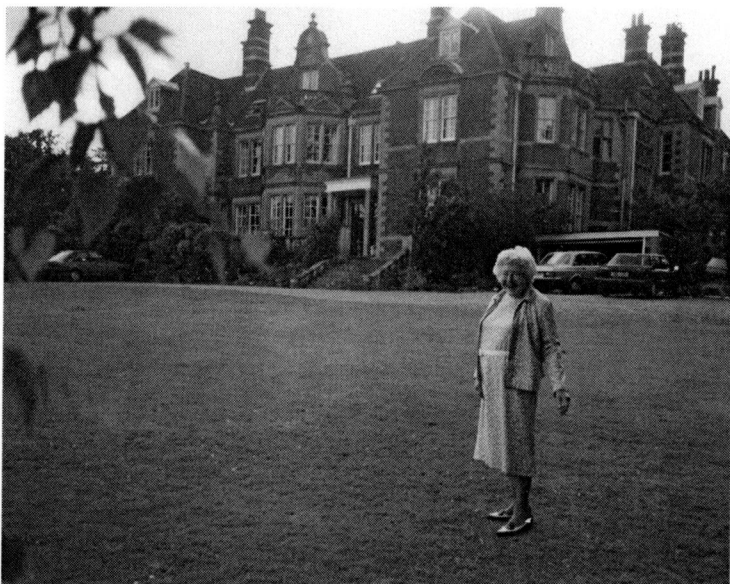

*Alli's mum, Letty, in front of The Terrace House. 1990*

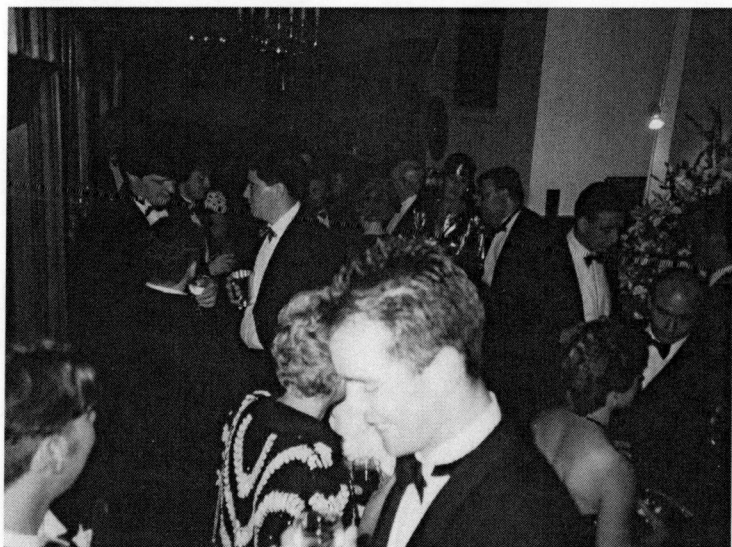

*The Terrace House, a real party house. Penny's 21st Birthday.*
*December 1990*

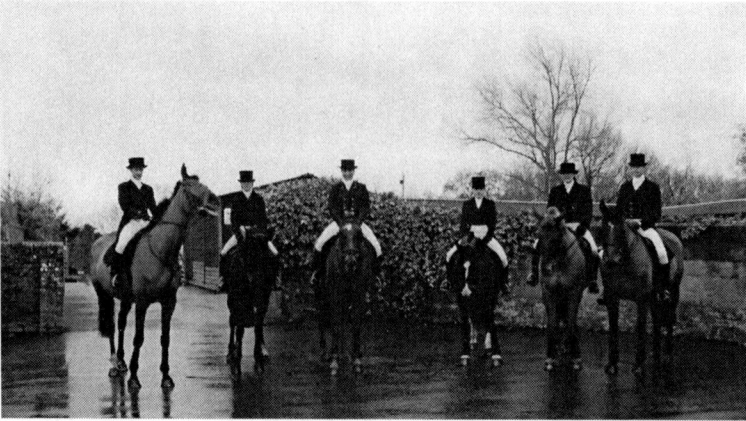

*Tish, Lucy, Natalie, Lauren, Caly & James at Alli's Funeral.*
*November 2003*

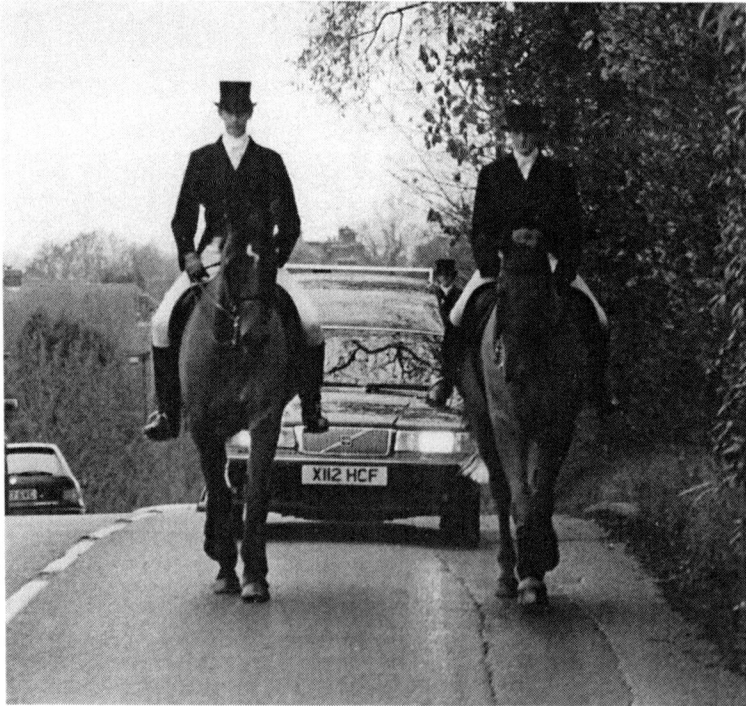

*James & Caly leading the cortege at Alli's Funeral.*
*November 2003*

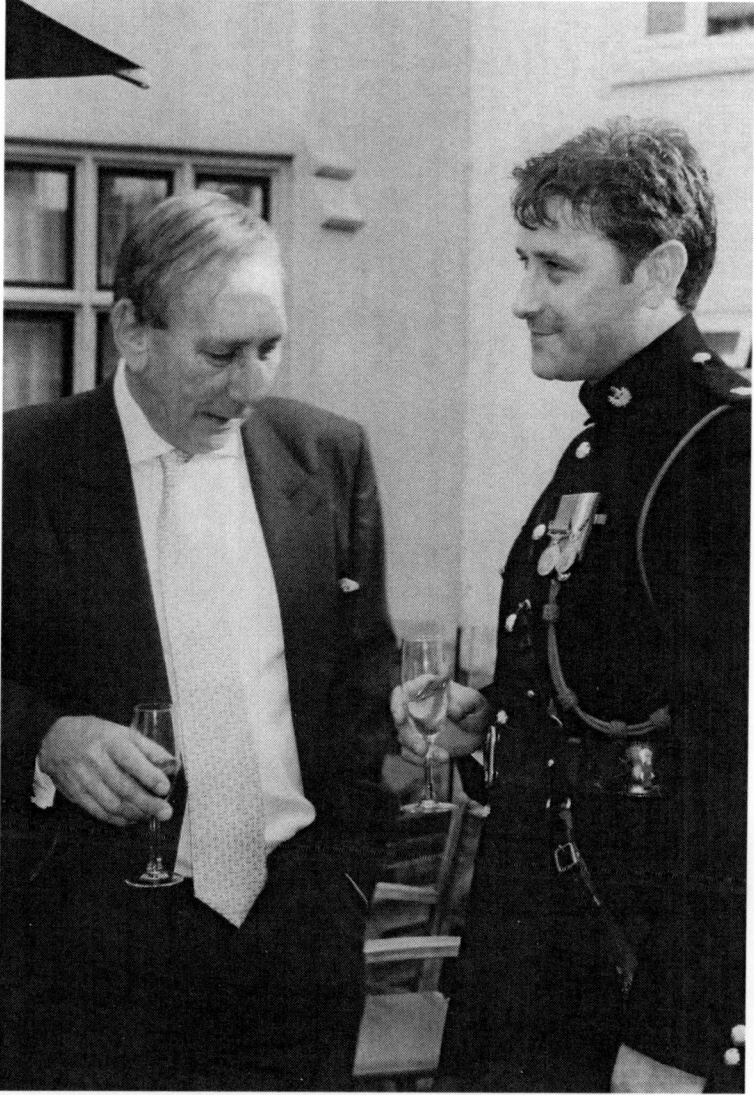

*A proud father outranked by his son Major Duncan Sangster. 2005*

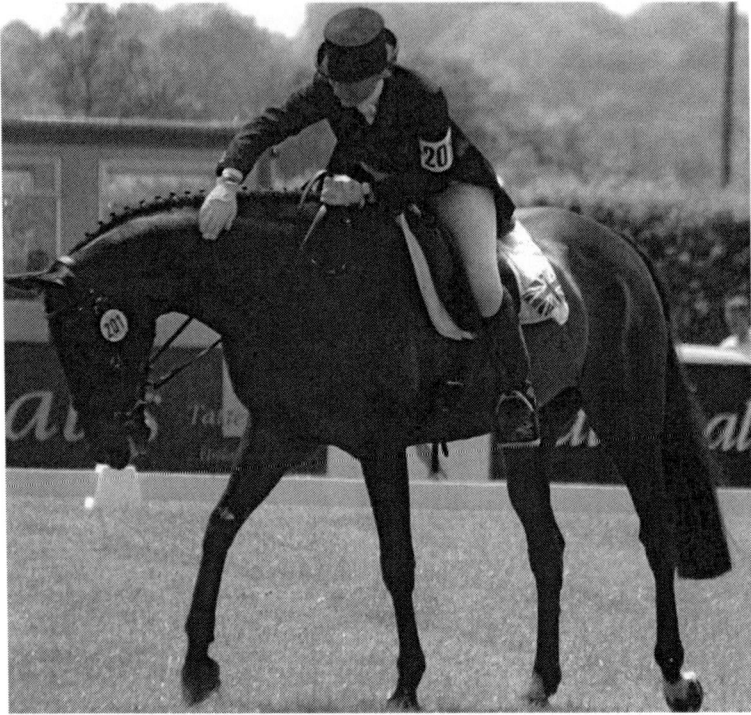

*Penny after the dressage at Tattersalls, Ireland CCI\*\*\**
*World Cup Qualifier. 2009*

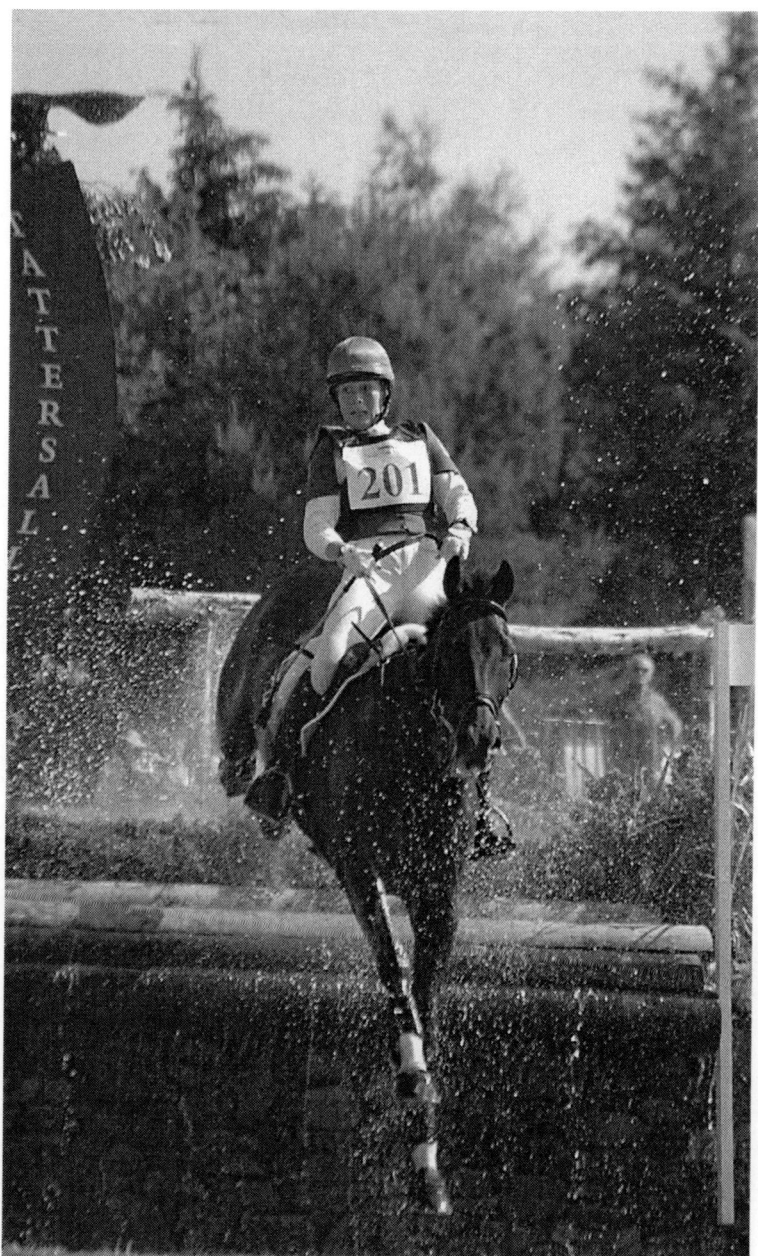

*Penny on the cross-country at Tattersalls, Ireland CCI\*\*\* World Cup Qualifier. 2009*

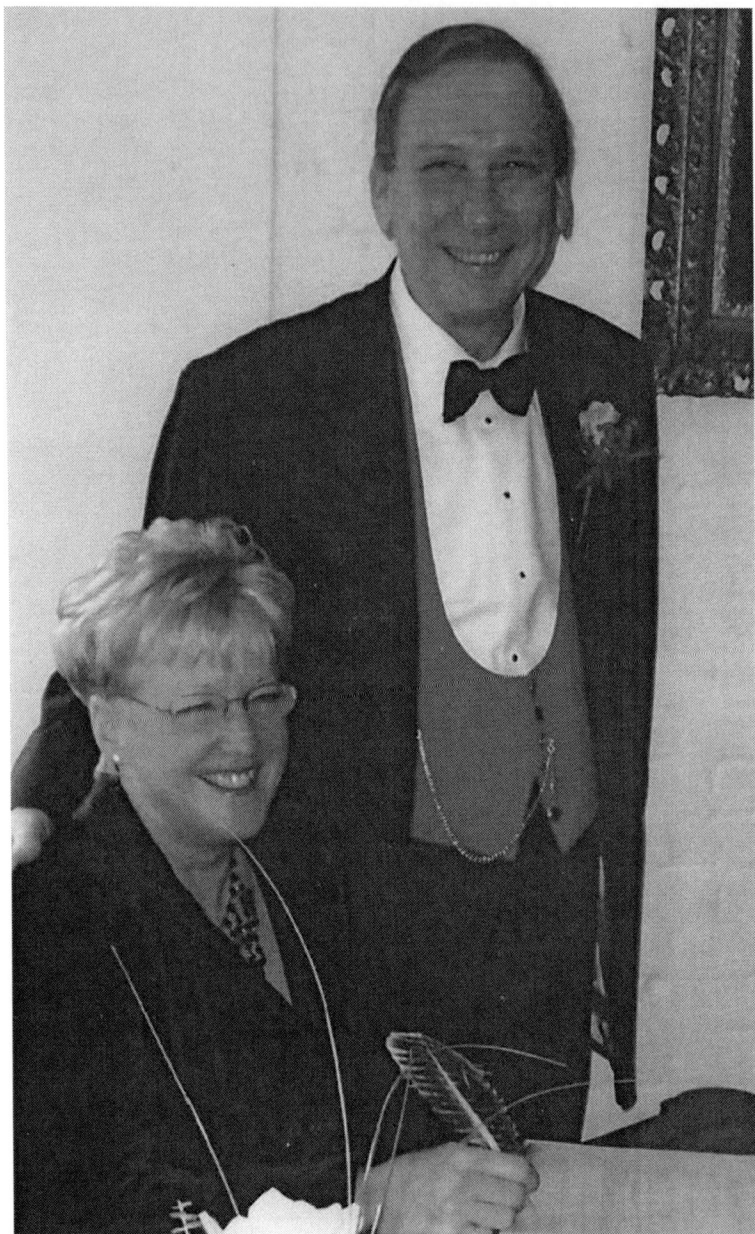

*Linda & Me 6th January 2005*

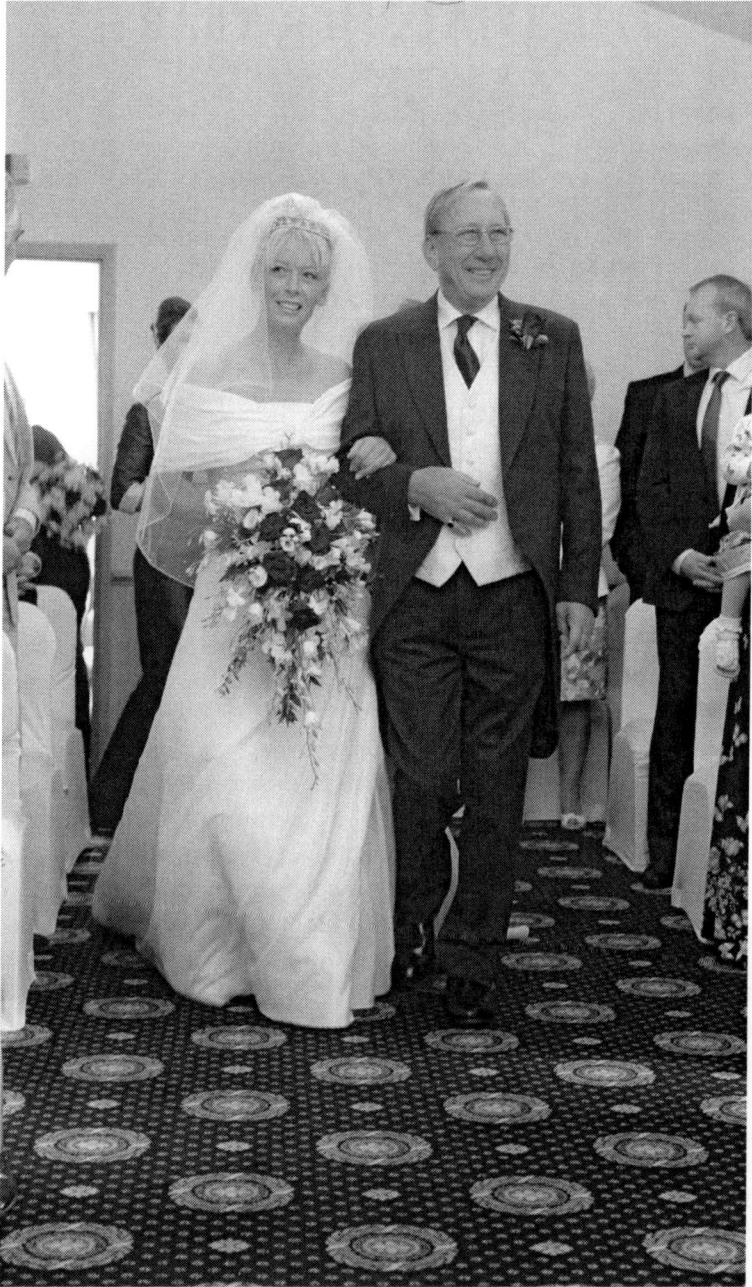

*Penny's wedding 25th June 2011*

# Chapter 8
# THE THATCHER YEARS

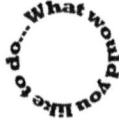

I had difficulty in deciding on a title for this chapter but The Thatcher Years seems right; everyone knows that the 1980s were just that.

However, Margaret Thatcher herself did not always get it right. In 1974 in an interview with the *Liverpool Post* she said:

> It will be years before a woman either leads the party or becomes Prime Minister. I certainly do not expect to see it happen in my time.

How wrong she was!

Perhaps this is an appropriate point for me to explain the sort of person PNS is and the influence he has had on me as a boss and friend.

First and foremost, PNS was Margaret Thatcher's number one admirer—he even once went on a trade mission flying to Italy with her. We could not help calling PNS a 'captain of British industry'. PNS is a loud man—by this I mean in voice. He puts this down to his having to stand up for himself when a schoolboy; as I have previously said, I believe it has more to do with his nature and inherited genes. His intellect is exceptional: two honours degrees from Cambridge, a chartered accountant and a Fellow of the Chartered Insurance Institute. He is also full of energy, enthusiasm and inspiration. Put these qualities together and the result can be extremely frightening to mere mortals like me. However, PNS did not like yes men and appreciated anyone who would stand up for himself. On occasions I would to say to him quietly 'Peter, you're wrong', and he would usually stop and listen, and more often than not modify his views and subsequent decisions. However, the few occasions when PNS was unusually quiet were the most dangerous times, since this meant that for some reason he was extremely angry. Those of us who were wise would keep a low profile on those occasions and look out for whatever wrath he was to deliver on whoever was the target.

On PNS's instructions I had helped Jim Doran, our new manager in Liverpool, to recruit the staff, although this had involved not much more than interviewing the three people whom Jim had 'poached' from Royal Insurance, and found and set up an ideal office. We managed to rent a nice, small, private office at the rear of what was the old Martins Bank head office, and which I remembered from when I had worked in that building 15 earlier and it was occupied by Cornhill Insurance Company. I organised golf days for the brokers, which PNS loved, and cocktail parties which were to become an annual feature for all our regional offices. I was able to get Bob Paisley (Liverpool FC manager at the time) to attend as the special guest for our opening cocktail party. This went down very well with the brokers.

At the beginning of February 1980 I spent a week helping them to understand our systems and procedures, and was able to stay with my parents. My father was not well. He had suffered from a bad cold and his breathing was extremely difficult. I persuaded him to let me call a doctor. Father was immediately admitted to hospital. I caught the Friday afternoon train back to Sussex.

Alli and I had decided to try to find a house with more land. We had an offer on our own house, so on that Saturday morning we went to see a cottage in the Ashdown Forest with ten acres of fields. When Alli and I got home, my mother phoned to say that Dad had died. On the Sunday I immediately caught a train back to Liverpool and my sister also came up from Somerset to comfort Mum and make the necessary arrangements for Dad's will and funeral. Brenda stayed with Mum and I again caught the Friday afternoon train back to Sussex. I remember that it started snowing. The funeral was to be the following Thursday. At the time, Brian Armstrong, the brother of Alli's sister-in-law, was staying with us and could look after Penny and Duncan overnight, and friends kindly agreed to take them to school and look after them after school until Brian returned from work while Alli and I were away in Liverpool. As I came out of the crematorium following Father's funeral service, Dad's neighbour approached me and said that the Sussex Police had been on the phone; that very morning our house had caught fire. Penny and Duncan were safe and staying with friends. Alli and I immediately returned to Sussex to find the whole of the upstairs of the house badly burnt by a fire in a gable roof. Most of the interior decoration was smoke-damaged and the downstairs, except the lounge, was soaked with the water used by the Fire Brigade. The insurance claim came to over £20,0000; I was the first member of staff to appear on the company's large-loss list!

It was a very traumatic experience, but if there was a good side to this major upset it is that, as an insurance man, I now have both empathy and sympathy with anyone who suffers similar circumstances. It is important for insurers to provide a claims service which is as efficient and trouble-free as possible, which is not always the case. This is a principle that I always adhered to when I became directly involved in underwriting.

We set to rescuing what belongings had survived the fire, smoke and water damage and stored them in the lounge, in which Penny and Duncan were able to have a bed each. I borrowed a caravan from my brother-in-law and Alli and I slept in the caravan, which we also used for cooking and eating for the next six months that it took for the re-building works to be completed. The couple who wanted to buy our house were in no hurry and were prepared to wait while the house was repaired. This meant that the entire house could be re-decorated to their fashion. The cottage in the Ashdown Forest that Alli and I wanted was the subject of an executor sale and the trustees were also happy to delay completion. So out of disaster came good, and by September 1980 we were in our new home with plenty of land for ponies and horses, much to the delight of Alli and Penny.

Duncan also enjoyed riding, but was much more interested in playing mini rugby. I was delighted to be able to train the young boys on Sunday mornings at East Grinstead Rugby Club. At the end-of-season barbecue and prize-giving in April 1981, Andy Ripley, who played for Roslyn Park and was a well-capped England and Lions Number 8, came to encourage the boys and present the awards. Five years later I was to meet Andy again, when I was able to persuade him to be our after-dinner speaker at a management conference I organised. We became good friends, and 15 years later he was very supportive to me as a non-executive director of my company. I will talk more about Andy later in the book, as he also was to be a great influence on me, and not just in my business life. Sadly, Andy died in June 2010 after a five-year fight with prostate cancer. During the last few months before he died I visited him at home on occasions and experienced how devastating the illness and the effect of the drugs can be in the later stages. One week after he died I was diagnosed with lung cancer, and the example he showed, and how he faced up to it and dealt with it, has been a huge inspiration to me in coming to terms and coping.

At work between 1980 and 1983 I was involved in recruiting management and staff to open new regional offices in Birmingham and

Bristol, and became more involved in regional business development. The insurance industry is a strange one in that, apart from a slight increase in claims during recessionary times, it does not seem to suffer from a downturn when the rest of the economy is suffering. It does have its bad times, but they are generally self-inflicted by too much capacity, competition and greed. Major disasters like Piper Alpha, Opren and large windstorms and hurricanes also take their toll. One underwriter had once described underwriting to me as when greed overcomes fear.

The early 1980s were a time of severe competition and stupidity in reducing rates, and particularly UK property and liability underwriting results were becoming unsustainable as a result. PNS had taken over as managing director and chief executive of the company and in 1983 our parent company, Ennia NV, merged with another large Dutch insurance group and the new group was re-launched as AEGON. We in the UK took on the new group style and logo as part of a parent group, which had doubled in size.

Soon after this, the Dutch appointed a new director called Alan Halford to our UK Board to take responsibility for the regional offices and UK business development. Alan had spent his life as an inspector in business development rather than in technical underwriting. He was a bit of a playboy character, and this did not go down well with some of the regional office managers, who had high standards of underwriting. Then in September 1984 Jim Doran, who was our manager in Liverpool, unexpectedly resigned and left, partly because he could not get on with Alan Halford. While Jim was working his notice, Alan had a pulmonary embolism and died suddenly of a heart attack. This may seem sad, but at the time he was on a week's holiday, having told the company that he was going to Spain with some friends to play golf and his wife that he was away in Holland on business. In fact he died at 7.30 in the morning in bed in a hotel room on the Costa Brava with his 'fancy woman'. PNS took back responsibility for the regional offices and, because of the uncertainty in the company's underwriting results, did not feel that it was the best time to recruit an outsider to fill the position. He asked me if I would take over and run the Liverpool office for the time being.

Again I was faced with that question WHAT WOULD YOU LIKE TO DO?

This time I had no hesitation. I grabbed the opportunity with both hands, because at long last it was my chance to get involved with underwriting and the front-line trading of the company.

Liverpool Office had an assistant manager called Tony Docherty who was, understandably, a bit upset at not having been appointed manager. PNS counselled Tony carefully and, rather like what Tony Blair said later to Gordon Brown when Gordon felt he should be in charge of New Labour, told Tony that he wanted him to help me take over as manager and 'learn the trade' before moving me back to London to a more senior post, which would only be for a short time. PNS promised Tony that he would then succeed me in the position of manager. Tony reluctantly accepted this, and when I arrived he rather bluntly asked me what I was going to do as his new manager. I immediately suggested that for the first 12 months I would handle all the renewals and would leave Tony to concentrate on quoting and developing new business, which is the more exciting aspect of underwriting. Tony was happy with this plan, and it gave me the opportunity to go through every file and learn the ropes from what had gone before. Tony and I developed a wonderful relationship, where he was happy to be the expert and let me get on as the person to deal with the more 'political' aspects of management. He was very supportive and helped me enormously, and we have remained friends ever since. As a new man in the local market I could get away with making unpleasant decisions and push up rates in an attempt to improve the underwriting results of the office, which had not been very good. Tony and I became good friends and work colleagues, and I am very grateful for the support he gave me over those important two years of 1986 and 1987.

The office in Liverpool covered the whole of the North of England and Scotland. We had a reasonable account with a the Glasgow branch of a national broker called Stewart Wrightson, later to become part of the Willis Group, and the director we dealt with was Douglas Eliot. I went to Scotland to meet Douglas in 1986 and not only did we develop some profitable business together, but also Douglas became and still is a very close friend. Many, like me as a teenager, may consider that insurance is a boring, desk-based job, but in fact it is a fascinating business with many interesting and amusing experiences. I recall some of these in the business which I underwrote through Douglas.

I underwrote a scheme for the Scottish Licensed Trade Association which had about 4000 members, hotels, bars and restaurants in Scotland. On one occasion, Douglas phoned me at 4.30 on a Friday afternoon and asked me to cover a 'hydroponicum' in the Summer

Isles Hotel. What on earth was a hydroponicum, and how do you rate the risk, I asked myself. Apparently it was a large greenhouse in which the hotel grew vegetables and fruit where the roots were suspended in flowing water rather than in soil. I agreed to cover the risk as an extension to the main buildings of the hotel. Then a bar in Glasgow called The 39 Steps had a very extensive stock of malt whiskies, and one of the staff dropped a bottle of 50-year-old Macallan; the bottle did not break but there was a crack in its neck. Macallan inspected the bottle and decanted the nectar, which was judged OK for consumption but not for sale. We had to pay a claim of £1000 for the whisky and Douglas bought the salvage, which he gave to me on my next trip to Glasgow. This has long since been consumed, but I kept it for special occasions and friends who appreciated both the story and the whisky.

I also underwrote the public liability insurance for the plant hire group Hewden Stewart. Just before Christmas 1968, a company was doing repair work on an American airbase in eastern England and had hired plant from Hewden Stewart. A foreman had instructed one of his operatives to take a hired tractor and power-take-off and dig up an old concrete base. As the operative started his pneumatic drill it was whipped from his hands and he looked round to see the tractor unit motoring across the grass only to crash into a top-secret American spy-plane which was taxiing on the runway. Over $2million damage. The operative was taken in and questioned for 36 hours by the CIA, and our loss adjusters were not allowed on site or to take any photographs of the damage. For some reason, thankfully, the US Government never did lodge a claim against us. Another time, Hewden Stewart had hired a tower crane to contractors building offices in Lower Thames Street in London, and the crane suddenly collapsed and fell on a Christopher Wren church, causing over £2 million damage to the roof. It turned out that the fixing bolts for the base of the crane had been supplied by a small engineering company to a wrong specification, so yet again no claim was made against us. Finally, I recall that we insured a small engineering company in Glasgow and again, at 4.30 one Friday afternoon, Douglas phoned me and told me that there had been a fatality when a coupling on an overhead gantry had snapped and a ton of machinery had fallen on a worker, who had been killed. I immediately phoned my claims manager and told him, and his immediate response was to ask whether the deceased was wearing a hard hat at the time—claims managers have a rather sordid sense of humour! It later transpired that the unlucky victim had no dependents, his children having grown up and become financially independent, and that at 2.00 pm on the very afternoon of the accident his divorced wife had remarried. This sad story meant that the fatality claim cost us only a fraction of what it could have been in other circumstances. Someone once asked:

> Never mind if he is a good underwriter, is he a lucky underwriter?

I have had my share of luck.

In the late 1980s Douglas invited me to Glasgow as his guest at Erskine Golf Club Burn's Night Dinners. These were truly memorable, as no wine was consumed. Instead each table had copious bottles of whisky and the next morning I had to face a full Scottish fried breakfast which Douglas's lovely wife Rosemary cooked for me before I caught my flight home. So I am grateful to Douglas for some memorable experiences, not just in business but also in monumental hangovers! Like a true lifetime friend, he still phones me regularly to see how I am getting on, and we meet at least once each year to play golf, dine and reminisce which, because we live so far apart, is frequently in the Algarve, where Douglas has a villa and Linda and I often go for golfing holidays.

In the meantime, the Dutch head-hunted and appointed yet another new director, David Pye, to take charge of UK underwriting and regional offices. If ever there was a chalk and cheese situation, Alan Halford and David Pye epitomised it. David had an impressive CV, being a Fellow of the Chartered Insurance Institute and a graduate, and had an MBA. What he had in letters after his name he totally lacked in business acumen. David was not a risk taker so how he ever got into underwriting I will never understand. It is interesting to note that he had never stayed in a company for more than five years, and all his promotions were by changing jobs—a clear indication that wherever he had worked he had been sussed out as very impressive on paper and at interview but not very effective in practice. David became even more unpopular with the regional managers and staff than Alan Halford had been, but for totally different reasons. He tended to ignore me, since he found it frustrating to have to cope with my reasoning and constant challenges of his decisions. The other regional managers just paid David lip service, ignored him and got on with things in their own way.

In the mid-1980s underwriting results in the whole world-wide insurance industry were not very impressive, and the first to react to this were the reinsurance companies (most of which were European, led by the Swiss, Germans and French), which withdrew the support that the direct insurance industry relies on in a wholesale manner. Relatively small insurance companies relied on the support of reinsurance capacity to be able to write risks which had a reasonable level of sums insured, or had either to decline business at renewal or find alternative ways and markets to replace their lost capacity. I discovered that reinsurers were prepared to support specialised areas of underwriting which were simple to understand and control, and which were less susceptible to the risk of unknown accumulation and loss aggregation. Off my own bat, I therefore set about placing a specific quota share treaty for regional office business. With the help of a very competent reinsurance broker called Colin Sampson I succeeded in doing well enough to enable us to renew the bulk of our existing good business against an ambitious promise to increase rates on average by 25%. I devised a system of recording a premium/rating comparison between expiry and renewal terms and set about the task, almost unsupported by our competitors and the brokers with whom we dealt. However, it did not take long for the rest of the market to cotton on to the fact that prices had to go up, and in my first full year of underwriting in 1986 I managed to achieve more than a 25% overall rate increase.

This, together with Tony Docherty's taking advantage of our competitors' inability to renew business, resulted in Liverpool Office increasing its book by 150% while returning healthy and profitable underwriting results. It also meant that we needed more staff and larger premises. I looked for a new office, and the bank offered to take back the lease on our existing office space. The directors were happy with the way things were going, but decided that Manchester rather than Liverpool was now the insurance centre of the North of England and that, with an opportunity to move office, it should be to Manchester. Now some of you may know about the rivalry, which almost borders on hatred, between Liverpool and Manchester; the staff, who were all Scousers, were absolutely mortified at the thought of moving the office 45 miles east of their beloved Liverpool.

When I first took over the Liverpool office I still had to oversee the administration and personnel work, which had become less of a burden because I had built up a department with very competent staff and had overcome the staff unrest and turnover that had existed in 1980 when I took over. I had almost worked myself out of a job. I flew to Manchester each Monday morning and back on Thursday evenings, and I stayed with Don and Gill, Alli's youngest brother and his wife, rather than experience hotel life, which I hated as a long-term form of existence. Friday was spent in the Edenbridge office dealing with staff and admin issues. It was a bit *déjà vu* but the reverse of 1968/69 when I was travelling in the opposite direction. Clearly this could not be a permanent arrangement, and the company agreed that I should relocate to the North West and relinquish my admin and personnel duties. In the summer of 1985 we sold our cottage in the Ashdown Forest and moved into a four-bedroom house in the Wirral with five acres and room to build a stable block, taking our ponies with us. Penny was 15 and a bit of a bolshie teenager. She did not want to move from Sussex to 'such a hell hole as Liverpool' and was just about to start her O Level year. I had personally experienced the upset of moving schools and syllabus in my own O Level year, so Alli and I agreed that she could stay during term time with Ben and Cherry Van Praagh, who were very good friends of ours, and come home for the holidays.

We were also concerned that the standard of schools near where we were moving was not as high as Sackville School in East Grinstead where Penny and Duncan had been for the past few years. As far as Duncan was concerned, Alli and I were even more concerned that he was being dragged down and was not doing very well academically. We were therefore glad of the opportunity to put him into the private education system. Following a short interview with John Gwilliam, who was the headmaster of Birkenhead School (a man of Welsh Chapel upbringing who in his younger days was an International Cap at Rugby for Wales and the British Lions), Duncan was accepted at Birkenhead and started in September 1986. I can only guess that Duncan impressed Mr Gwilliam by his rugby prowess rather than by answering questions relating to his intellect. This was an excellent move for Duncan, and he soon settled in, enjoying playing rugby and being in the Combined Cadet Force. He also made some good new friends and was soon much happier than he had been at Sackville. Penny came home for the Christmas holidays. Despite her age and attitude to parents, I think she had actually missed us. Because Duncan had made new friends, Penny was able to meet and make friends with other youngsters of her age, and she started to warm to our new home and began to think that Liverpool was not quite such a bad place as she had thought. Although I no longer had any relatives in the area, Alli's mum and three brothers and their families were scattered around, and it was wonderful to be able to spend time with them partying and for Penny and Duncan to get to know their aunts, uncles and cousins better. These were very happy days. But it was less than three years before I was to be asked to go back 'down South'.

In 1988 the company's treaty manager resigned and PNS asked me to return to London and take over his post. This involved underwriting the small inward treaty reinsurance and taking charge of placing the company's outward reinsurances. Treaty business is reinsurance which all insurance companies and Lloyd's syndicates place to give then capacity and to protect their account against an accumulation or aggregation of claims from one cause of loss (such as a hurricane or total loss of a property, ship or aeroplane). Treaties are underwritten on a portfolio of risks rather than on a risk-by-risk basis. This is a very different type of reinsurance, and is a world-wide market with several insurance companies specialising in this type of business. It is considerably less costly in administrative expenses to underwrite, so the margins can be less than those associated with direct insurance. Apart from being involved with placing our special regional office treaty, I had little knowledge of this area of insurance at that time. The job meant that I would have to work in London and Alli, Penny (who was now taking A Levels at Chester College) and Duncan (who had just finished O Levels and started his VIth Form A Level course) were very happy living in the Wirral.

Again I was faced with that question, WHAT WOULD YOU LIKE TO DO?

In terms of my career advancement I had no hesitation in wanting to take over the position, but I did not want to disrupt the family, and in particular Duncan's education and development. At a Birkenhead parent—teachers evening, Alli and I had been asked to speak with the headmaster. What on earth had Duncan been up to? John Gwilliam told us that he felt Duncan would struggle to obtain good A Level results but that he had shown qualities of leadership. We were being asked if we had a preferred route for him, whether the school should try and push him in his studies or encourage his leadership skills, which could distract him from his academic studies. We told John Gwilliam that we would be happy for the school to do whatever it thought was in Duncan's best interest, and I think he saw that we were more keen on developing his leadership. Over his last two years at Birkenhead Duncan became a prefect, head of his house and house rugby captain and a senior NCO in the CCF, but his A Level results were not very good and he was to struggle to get an offer to go to university. I asked PNS whether the company would agree to my family remaining in the Wirral for the next two years and pay the cost of my living in London in the meantime. This he agreed to, and for the next 21 months I was to stay during the week at the Cavalry and Guards Club and go home for the week-ends—once more a situation similar to that which Alli and I had experienced in 1968, but for a longer period.

Working in London with no daily family routine or commitments, as on the two previous occasion but for a longer period, meant that I arrived at the office early, worked later and frequently networked socially after work with market colleagues, all of which is very tiring. I needed the week-ends to recover. I would return, and all Alli wanted to do, having had to deal with two bolshie teenagers all week, was to go out for dinner and party. This life style continued for nearly two years and inevitably there was the risk that Alli and I would grow apart. That did not happen, and I will be ever grateful to Alli for the fact that all through our happy years together she always supported me in my career moves and the pressures of work. Most domestic difficulties arise where work and family interfere, and conflicts arise where the main breadwinner has to make a choice between work and home pressures. Thanks to Alli's wonderful support and love, I was never faced with this sort of dilemma.

The job of placing the company's reinsurance protections was truly interesting and rewarding. We conducted business with reinsurance companies as far away as Australia, Japan, Singapore, Russia, USA, Scandinavia and mainland Europe supporting our treaties. It would have been an impossible and expensive task to visit them all annually and answer their individual questions about our business. Each September a *rendezvous* of the world-wide reinsurance market took place in Monte Carlo, and in October another reinsurance meeting was held in Baden Baden in the Black Forest. These were hectic weeks of non-stop meetings and entertaining. They were made even better by the fact that PNS also attended, together with his wife Jean, and I was fortunate to be able to take Alli with me so that she could support me and have the pleasure of enjoying these exotic places.

At the end of 1989, David Pye, who was the director in charge of UK domestic fire and accident underwriting, resigned. PNS again took over the watch of the regional offices, and David's other duties were shared among the other directors. AEGON in Holland had recently appointed Kees Storm as the new CEO of the group, and there was much speculation and fear as to what the future might hold.

Fear is a little darkroom where negatives are developed.

This was written by Michael Pritchard, who was for over 20 years a researcher of photographic history and photographic technology, and spent more than 20 years as a Christie's photographic specialist. He has written and lectured extensively, and was awarded the Fellowship of the Royal Photographic Society for his work on the history of photography.

# Chapter 9
# MANAGEMENT

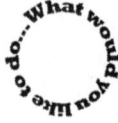

In my earlier years management was a subject which only subconsciously interested me. As I matured, the theory of management became a deep interest, and the practice of management has given me great personal satisfaction as well as more than occasional frustrations.

My view is that to be a manager you have to have the quality of leadership. The Army has always realised this. Leadership is **the** over-riding quality that the armed forces generally look for in selecting candidates for officer training. I firmly believe that without the ability to lead no-one can truly be a good manager, just a 'boss'. My favourite quotation on this subject comes from Russell H. Ewing.

> A boss creates fear, a leader confidence. A boss fixes blame, a leader corrects mistakes. A boss knows all, a leader asks questions. A boss makes work drudgery, a leader makes it interesting. A boss is interested in himself or herself, a leader is interested in the group.

There are many people who do not have the natural ability to lead, and thankfully most realise this. Others, sadly, do not, and in general do not make good managers. There is nothing wrong with a person who does not have leadership qualities, and very often such people have other wonderful talents and achieve great things in their lifetime.

There are many different styles of management. The one that I despise most is what I call Nazi management—management by fear. The worst example of this style of management I have personally experienced was when I worked at the Independent Insurance Company, which features in Chapter 10.

In 1980 I attended a training course entitled Development of Executives at Sundridge Management College and run by PA Management Consultants. I do not recall all that we were taught, but one of our lecturers was a man by the rather sinister name of Boris Gussman. In fact Boris was not at all sinister. He boasted that he was the first person in the UK to obtain a degree in Anthropology, and his understanding of human behaviour and what made people tick was both fascinating and instructive. One of the exercises we did was a personality test called the Kostic Profile. This involved answering a series of simple multiple choice questions about one's personal preferences, questions such as:

In your work, which gives you the most satisfaction?

A. Solving a problem?
B. Motivating others to work?
C. Completing a job?

Many of these questions were mixed and repeated, but asked in a slightly differently way and in a different context, such as:

What do you see as the best quality in a manager?

A. Setting out clear instructions for a task?
B. Setting targets for achievement?
C. Setting an example?

and:

If you were to apply for a new job, what would be your main reasons?

A. More freedom of decision?
B. More job satisfaction?
C. More responsibility?

In the test there were several hundred questions to be answered in a limited time so that the responses were intuitive. The answers were plotted on a circular graph, which gave a representation of your personality by showing high and low scores relating to your personality and character.

Two years after this I went for a job interview and was again subjected to a Kostic Profile test. The results were virtually identical to my previous test at Sundridge—I could not possibly have remembered the answers I had previously given. It may seem a bit sad, but I still have the chart of my original Kostic Profile and my main character traits show:

A. I am high in leadership
B. I am low in attention to detail
C. I have what is called a 'kettle lid' personality. I bottle up problems until they become urgent and then explode to solve them.

I cannot argue with these results!

In the early 1990s I organised a series of in-house management training courses for our middle management staff and I asked Boris to give some of the lectures. I engaged the Industrial Society, a training and advisory service greatly supported by some of the largest UK companies, for assistance in planning and organising the training. These courses were a resounding success, and a lot of up-and-coming junior managers benefited from Boris's brilliant teaching. A spin-off was that in 1994 I was asked by the Industrial Society to be an instructor and mentor at their Runge Effective Leadership course at Oxford University. It was a privilege to be asked. I was responsible for a small group of young managers from a variety of companies and industries who were presented with challenging management and leadership problems. It was a great stimulation to me, and I hope that my charges, whatever they are now doing, will also always look back on it as a wonderful experience.

During the early 1980s, as part of my job as admin and personnel manager, I also organised the annual company management week-ends. At the 1982 conference, each of the company's managers was asked to give a presentation on some aspect of his or her department's work. I decided to deal with the management aspects of being personnel manager. To illustrate this I gave a presentation of the organisation and management of an imaginary company called 'Any Old Insurance Company Limited'. I chose the managers of this company by their initials, which by some accident happened to be the same as those of my colleagues! This allowed me to describe some of the different ways in which people manage. The company was made up of the following management.

Dept. S. The manager was Mr 'All Good Workers'. This manager always praised his workers as the best. Occasionally they were not, so he would then get stuck in and rectify their errors so as to cover up for his staff's shortcomings.

Dept. R. The manager was Mr 'Menacing Staff'. This manager is a friendly man who enjoys the people who work for him. However, from time to time 'people' undergo a strange metamorphosis and turn into 'difficult staff', and he could not cope with this and always needed the support of the personnel department to sort out the mess.

Dept. T. The manager was Mr 'Rabble Just Shut-up'. This manager was technically very competent but would sit in his office with the door shut and get on with his work, and expected his staff to do the same.

Dept. C. The manager was Mr 'Workers Can't Manage'. This manager was always complaining that his staff were overworked and saw the only solution as recruiting more staff to cope with the workload. His department, coincidentally, also had the highest average overtime per person of the company.

Dept. P. The manager was Mr 'Jungle-bunnies Witless, Efficient Caucasians'. This was the 'black and white' manager. Things were only ever right or wrong, good or bad, positive or negative, etc., and there was never anything in life in between. Invariably, right, good and positive were only those things that he agreed with and would support, and conversely . . . !

The director responsible for staff was Mr 'Reward or Sack the Workers' who believed that everyone should be paid more but if they did not perform they should be mercilessly sacked. In his view, everyone from time to time 'did not perform' so there was a real risk of the personnel department having to spend all its time sacking, then recruiting and training.

The Managing Director was Mr 'Pay No Salary-rises'.
To this last character, I remember PNS bellowing out 'that's not true'. Of course none of it was completely true, but I was able to illustrate how different managers had different approaches to

managing staff. I concluded with the personnel manager, who was called Mr 'Poor Bloody Sod', because he sat in the middle of this maelstrom of different management styles having to sort out the resulting mess.

Some of my colleagues found my presentation highly entertaining. Sadly, there was one who was so upset at what I had said that on the following Monday he sought legal advice to consider suing me for defamation. He was politely advised to forget about it and get on with his work!

In Chapter 6, I talked about various women in my life, but it would be remiss of me not to give my views about women in management. I am not a woman hater or misogynist (at least I do not think I am) but I realise that some of my views, which are based on experience as well as being my personal opinion, may not go down well with some of my readers. I will take that risk.

As I have mentioned, I believe that one of the fundamental qualities of a good manager is leadership. As a generalisation, I also believe that the fairer sex were 'not made' to be leaders since leadership sometimes demands a degree of aggression and dispassion is necessary for leadership to manifest itself. Women have great qualities which generally speaking men do not possess. They include the ability to multi-task (which is a great ability, but can have the disadvantage of distracting focus from the immediate problem to be solved) and a natural protective instinct which, accompanied by their greater sense of compassion and love, can result in decisions which may not be for the right reasons or for the benefit of the group as a whole.

Another belief which I have which will anger some is that, while I agree with the principle of equal opportunities for all, regardless of sex, colour, creed or any other way in which someone is different from others, I have always refused to accept that this means there should be equal representation. At a recent meeting of the trustees of a charity of which I was chairman, we were discussing prospective new trustees to fill vacancies arising from the retirement of trustees by rotation as required by the articles of association. The former 12 trustees consisted of five women and seven men, and the new Board of trustees would have fewer women and more men going forward. One of the male trustees raised the question of whether we should seek more women to become trustees to 'correct any imbalance'. My response was a little blunt. I made it quite clear that, as trustees, we had an over-riding prudential duty to ensure that the Board consisted of as many people as possible who could provide the expertise necessary to direct the charity, and not to fill vacancies with people because of their gender or any other unique 'difference' in order to be seen as 'politically correct'.

I have no problems with women in business or in management so long as, like anyone else, they are capable of doing the job. I do have problems with appointing people who are not capable of managing just to satisfy some groups in society, whether minority or not, whether physically different or not, just so that we can achieve 'proportional representation'! To put it in a more cruel but illustrative way, sadly there are people who have learning disabilities and they form a 'group' just as much as men, women, black or white people are part of a 'group'. Should we have proportional representation in management of people with a learning disability when clearly, because of their disability, they are not capable of performing the job? Another example is the nursing and care professions. Historically women have predominantly occupied posts in these professions. This is not because men do not want to enter these professions; in recent years more men have done so than in the past. It is because women generally have talents and characteristics which are better suited to nursing and care. The same applies to any other jobs; management is not a status or class but a job, the same as any other.

Harriet Harman (or as one of my friends calls her, Harriet Harperson!) professes equal representation. I say, by all means equal opportunity, but by no means guaranteed equal representation if it means that people will be appointed to jobs that they are not capable of performing.

Another great attitude to management is expressed in the Peter Principle which states:

Everyone is promoted to his level of incompetence.

Sadly, this has often been true when people have been promoted just because they are good at their job and show ambition, but without considering whether or not they are capable of doing a more senior or managerial job. I have seen this so many times in my life, and inevitably it has resulted in the over-promoted person not performing, not being happy and wishing that they were doing their old job, and it all ending in tears one way or another.

I will end this chapter on my views of management with a quotation for those who seek to be a better manager. It is from The Duke of Wellington who, when on his deathbed a friend asked:

> Sir, you have been a great leader, soldier and an eminent politician and have achieved more than most people do in their lifetime. What do you most regret?,

replied:

> I regret that I did not praise others more.

## Chapter 10
# I MADE IT

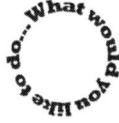

In January 1990 Kees Storm attended a board meeting in London and following this I was called into PNS's office and told that I had been appointed a director of AEGON Insurance Company (UK) Limited (AIC) and was to take over Board responsibility for the UK regional offices, as well as for reinsurance and staff and personnel.

This was the first time in my life that I had come to a major crossroad but was not faced with that question WHAT WOULD YOU LIKE TO DO? I had been told what I would do, and I liked it. I had a feeling of real success that I had achieved a long-held ambition to be a director of AIC.

Chet Atkins, a very gifted guitarist who created the Nashville Sound and of whom I was a great fan during my late teens, surprisingly best described my feelings about my promotion when he said:

> A long apprenticeship is the most logical way to success. The only alternative is overnight stardom, but I can't give you a formula for that.

For the first time I now believed that I could truly be in control of my life, or at least my working life. What a stupid and arrogant opinion that was!

In 1989, AIC had taken a minority trade investment in a small Lloyd's Broker called P S Mosse and Partners, and I had been appointed to the Board as a non-executive director. I was now a director of both Insurance Company and a Lloyd's Broker. This was not uncommon then, but today the Financial Services Authority would probably look on it with some concern about a potential conflict of interest in being a director of both an insurance company and an insurance broker. In addition my son, Duncan, worked for Mosse as a trainee broker. I have never had any problem with nepotism so long as it does not result in favouritism, and I think that Duncan will agree that, rather than benefiting from it, he had to try harder to prove himself.

The next three and a half years were to be some of the most exiting and enjoyable of my working life. Kees Storm (group CEO of AEGON) was a dynamic man and a natural leader who, like me, enjoyed challenges and competition in business. I immediately set about setting budgetary targets for each of my regional offices for expense control, premium income and underwriting profitability, which I coupled with a competition for the best regional office of the year. I also introduced regular managerial meetings to discuss issues of common interest and to ensure that all my managers were kept up to date with what was happening in other divisions of the company. I also made sure that I visited each office regularly to meet and talk to all the staff.

Until the beginning of 1990, for nearly two years I had lived during the week at the Cavalry and Guards Club in London and returned to my family in the Wirral at week-ends. This was clearly unsatisfactory, since Duncan was now living and working in London and Penny had gone to work as a groom in Karen Straker's eventing yard in North Yorkshire. I was based in Edenbridge in Kent with regular visits to London for meetings, while Alli was alone during the week in the Wirral. We had to move back to the South East. By chance, a business associate mentioned that he wanted to sell his house in Coleman's Hatch on the edge of the Ashdown Forest, where Alli and I had lived immediately before moving to the North West in 1986. This was The Terrace House, which was the larger portion of a Victorian mansion with over 9000 square feet of accommodation which, as well a very large drawing room and dining room, included a hall which was 48 feet long and 12 feet wide, from which a large staircase rose to the first and second floors where there were seven bedrooms with five bathrooms. Alli and I both knew the house from when we had previously lived in the village, and I knew that we could not afford the price that was being asked. Unexpectedly, the owner agreed to sell me the house at the maximum we could afford to pay, which was below the asking price. We rapidly agreed, completed the purchase and moved back down to East Sussex. This was the first and only time that Alli did not even go and look at a house before we agreed to buy it.

At the end of 1990 Penny moved back home and worked in a local show-jumping yard and Duncan moved in, commuting to London each day. The Terrace House was a wonderful party house and over the next five years we celebrated Penny's and Duncan's

21st birthdays, as well as our 25th wedding anniversary, in lavish style. We could comfortably accommodate more than 150 guests in the house at a party without any risk of overcrowding. Penny's and Duncan's friends came regularly to stay for week-ends and holidays. On Super Bowl night each year, Duncan had several mates round to watch the American football until the early hours of the morning and played mess rugby in the hall, on one occasion breaking one of my ribs in a crunching tackle against a radiator! In 1992 Alli first had a heart condition and was hospitalised for three weeks. Apart from this worry, the five years we lived there were full of fun and parties to a standard that we would never have dreamed we would be privileged to experience. We also used the house for junior management training courses for staff. Life was going very well.

In Board meetings I was constantly having to defend the fact that regional office business was more labour-intensive and had higher unit costs per pound of premium income than the relatively low production cost of London Market business. Despite this, my fellow directors continued to give me the support, encouragement and autonomy to expand the business. Between 1990 and the end of 1993 the regional office business grew from a premium income of less than £10 million to more than £70 million, with very positive underwriting results and a drastically reduced expense-to-premium ratio. This was not without its problems.

I have mentioned my involvement as a non-executive director of the Lloyd's Broker P S Mosse & Partners Limited (Mosse) in which AIC had a trade investment. This led to one of the most difficult experiences of my working life. In early December 1993, John Shepherd, the managing director of Mosse, phoned me and asked for a meeting later that morning. John, together with another director and the accountant, came to my office and told me that there appeared to be a 'hole' in the IBA (insurance escrow accounts which held underwriters' premiums) of about £750,000 and that cover notes had been issued when reinsurance cover had not actually been placed. It appeared that the misdemeanours fell fully at the feet of the chairman and chief executive, Alan Collins, and he asked me for my help. I agreed, and went to see Alan, who at first denied all knowledge but, when presented with some evidence, admitted that he had signed the wrong cover notes but still denied all knowledge of the missing insurance premium moneys. This was a serious matter, and at the request of the directors I suspended Alan and took over as chairman of the Board until the matter had been fully investigated. It soon became apparent that insurers' funds had been diverted, and it seemed that they had been paid to a Lichtenstein bank from which we could get no information.

The outcome was that Mosse was insolvent, and I immediately called in the Lloyds' Brokers Department and handed over the chequebooks for the IBA bank accounts. I asked my old friend Tim Wells for advice, and together we appointed an insolvency practitioner and spent many nights burning the midnight candle trying to construct a rescue package. All this was of no avail, and Mosse had to be put into liquidation and all the staff (including my son) made immediately redundant with no compensation. Allan Collins was later disciplined by being expelled for life from the Lloyd's insurance market and fined £25,000 for fraudulently issuing cover notes, but the missing insurance funds were never pursued by either the liquidator or the police, so no criminal charges were brought against him. For me, it was a traumatic and worrying experience, especially having to make many honest and innocent workers redundant just before Christmas, even though many were able to secure new jobs on the basis of their experience and contacts. In many ways it helped me to be even more vigilant and determined to act in a totally proper and honest manner in business.

In October 2003 we were told by Holland that in a review of the Group's long-term structure, AIC did not 'fit in with the Group's strategy'. This was partly because the AEGON Group was 90% life and health business and, of the 10% non-life, half was Dutch domestic business which for 'political reasons' they had to retain, and the other half was AIC. In the early 1990s the London Market, particularly Lloyd's, had problems in the run off old years (that is the settlement of long tail claims on old policies covering such industrial diseases as asbestosis) and had transferred it to a new reinsurance vehicle. This was a cause of rumours in the international financial markets, and the institutional investors and stock market advisers to the Group were expressing worries about the London Market operation and whether some new horror story would come out of that. This was having a negative effect on the Group share price. In the UK we knew that we were a well-reserved and healthy operation and had contributed considerable profits over the past five years. Our Dutch colleagues said that they were not in a hurry to dispose of us, and in November 2003 it was agreed that we could work towards putting together a management buy-out.

We arranged for Watsons to carry out an actuarial audit of the company's technical insurance reserves and we approached Lazards to assist us and advise on finding an MBO. These arrangements, as it turned out, were to be more of a hindrance than a help to our achieving our objective.

Watsons produced their actuarial audit in February 2004 and presented it in draft to the directors and our Dutch colleagues at a meeting in The Hague. It was the first time that I had been exposed to actuaries and the actuarial approach to reserving and probabilities. It seems that actuaries, unlike business entrepreneurs, are totally incapable of taking any risks or giving a reasoned prediction without qualifying it and using figures 'for illustrative purposes'. In our case, Watsons found that our reserving was adequate (and in some areas more than adequate), with the possible exception of the long tail professional indemnity class about which they said that their predictions could be inaccurate by as much as a factor of 10. This was a bit like shooting themselves in the foot, and we asked exactly what their advice was actually worth! Rather than providing some comfort, it made the Dutch even more nervous about the future of AIC. Following this I wrote a memo to the Board in which I stated that, if Watson's worst-case scenario were to come to pass, it would not just be a problem for the company but would probably be Armageddon for the whole international insurance market. At the bottom I put a footnote stating that I used the word 'Armageddon' for illustrative purposes only. The actuaries did not appreciate my sense of humour!

I had taken some action towards tidying up the regional office business to make the financing of an MBO attractive, and had taken the painful decision to close our Southampton office to make cost savings without affecting the business, since it could be transferred to Bristol and south east offices without any material detrimental effect. However, in April 2004 it came to light that one of my fellow directors, who was responsible for London Market business (and who I had previously said I suspected had lied and was withholding information from the Board), had not disclosed a large number of claims advised on a professional indemnity cover for solicitors.

I have always thought that lying is a drug. You start off with a little 'fib' which gives you butterflies in your stomach, and if you get away with it the next 'untruth' is a bit bigger and so on to the extent that there is some sort of 'buzz' from lying.

My fellow director resigned, and I was put in charge of London Market UK property and liability business as well as regional offices, then controlling 80 staff and an expense budget of £5 million and premium income in excess of £100 million. Some senior managers under my control were unhappy, but I rose to the challenge and won their respect when they realised that I did not want to interfere with the underwriting but help them to develop new opportunities in both their career aspirations and business development. This was a very hectic but rewarding few months, as all the Board tried to get to grips with tidying up old problems in anticipation of negotiating a management buy-out of our company from the AEGON Group.

Unknown to us, Lazards (whom we had approached for possible advice) were also advisers to Independent Insurance Company. I would not for one minute suggest that Lazards did not strictly observe a Chinese Walls policy, so I accepted as a coincidence that in August we were told by the Dutch that they had agreed to sell the AIC business to Independent and that, except for a few staff who would be retained to run off the old AIC business, AIC employees would be transferring to Independent. I was told that my three fellow directors would stay with the run off but that I would be joining Independent.

I did not have a liking for Michael Bright (CEO of Independent) or his reputation of being ruthless in the way he managed and ran a business.

This was my biggest nightmare.

In 1986 when I was running Liverpool Office, Adam Wilson and I were asked to carry out a confidential investigation into Allstate Insurance Company based in Sale, Cheshire. Allstate was the UK subsidiary of the large Allstate USA insurance group which had decided that they wished to dispose of the UK direct insurance company. Adam and I spent most of our time with one of Allstate's accountants, Dennis Lomas. Dennis was a nice, helpful man, but we both felt that he was more of a yes man than a strong manager. Allstate had computer underwriting systems, underwriting expertise and distribution channels that AIC lacked, but their management accounting and reserving techniques were well behind those which we had developed at AIC. Allstate UK was a company of similar size to AIC, but had the expertise and underwrote a motor account and had established regional offices in the UK, which AIC at that time lacked. AIC was stronger in the London Market business than

Allstate. This was thus a great opportunity to acquire a business with both synergy and strengths which would mean AIC doubling in size, resulting in real growth in premium income, distribution channels and market presence, coupled with improved expense ratios. Adam and I wrote a report to the AIC Board recommending that we make an offer of £6 million to acquire Allstate. The directors accepted this and tendered an offer to Allstate USA. We heard nothing for a few weeks until it was announced in the financial press that Allstate was being sold for £6.5 million to a newly established insurance group called New Scotland, which later changed its name to Independent Insurance Company Limited and was to be headed by Michael Bright as CEO.

We felt that we had been used just to fix a price for an already done deal.

When I was told by our Dutch masters that I would be joining Independent, I pointed out that, as a director, unlike the staff I did not fall under the Transfer of Undertakings Regulations that applied to takeovers, and that I would therefore not automatically be joining Independent. I asked for a severance package which reflected the seniority of my position and length of service. This they agreed to, and offered me a package equivalent to twice my salary and anticipated bonus plus a generous transfer of my pension rights to a personal pension plan.

I was immediately summoned by Michael Bright, who was at the time on holiday, to visit him in his apartment near Malaga in Spain. I flew to Spain where Michael told me that, while he would not take me on as a director of Independent, he needed my support to help integrate the AIC business and staff, and offered me a two-year contract as a senior manager to assist him personally in this task at an increased salary, after which he would offer me a permanent position at Independent. If I decided not to accept this, he would honour whatever severance package AEGON were offering based on my enhanced salary and bonus prospects in two years' time.

Here we go again! I was faced with that awful question: WHAT WOULD YOU LIKE TO DO?

I did not want to move to Independent, and after a lot of heart searching and the invaluable support of my wife, Alli, I decided that I had a duty of loyalty to support the AIC staff, who I knew would find the transfer difficult, and for the only time in my life I decided to do what I would NOT like to do and accepted Michael Bright's offer.

On reflection, I now believe that this decision and the experience of working for Independent for the next two years made me a better person and was fundamental in making me more tolerant of others. I now know that at some time in your life you should do what you do not want to do and face up to the challenges that this presents. It may be a very painful experience, but if approached with a positive and determined attitude it will change the way you perceive life and enhance your chances of future success.

So I started at Independent and it was soon apparent that my concern that the company was managed by fear was a reality.

The staff were generally paid above average market salaries so, if they left or were sacked (which to me seemed to happen all too frequently), they would have to accept a reduction in their standard of living. Staff would be at their desk at 7.00 am, not because they had work to do, but in case some senior manager or Michael Bright himself happened to check up on them. Michael was always an early starter but, unlike his staff, frequently took time off during the day to rest so that he could keep going into the evening, either with meetings or in parties which the staff who had worked all day were expected to attend and support. Michael liked yes-men and subservient people around him, and I was not surprised to find that Dennis Lomas, whom I had first met at Allstate in 1986, was now chief accountant and soon after was appointed financial director. Also, Michael Bright had morals that I found unacceptable. Having office affairs was a sure way to promotion, and it was no secret that Michael himself had a child by one of his own personal assistants and maintained (at the company's expense) a Brighton 'regional office' which was the home of his illegitimate child's mother, who remained on the payroll. During the three years that I worked for Independent, three staff out of some 1200 committed suicide.

To many of the AIC staff the new culture was stressful. Within three months of the merger, 30 of the AIC staff either had been sacked or had left. I tried as best I could to encourage those who were left, urging them to adapt to the new environment, and many did this successfully while others kept a low profile and accepted their lot until something better cropped up for them. It was not a happy time. During the first four weeks I was directed to visit all the regional offices and 'fly the flag', together with Philip Condon who was the underwriting director (later to be appointed deputy managing director) and Alan Clarke who was the personnel director (whom I had known in the early 1980s when he was personnel manager of Lombard and I was administration and personnel manager of AIC). I did this willingly because I saw it as an opportunity to support the AIC staff in the remote offices. First we went to the Bristol and Cardiff offices where the relatively few AIC staff seemed resigned to their fate and were moving forward. Then we drove to Manchester and the driver took us to the house of a lady who was the 'partner' of Philip Condon and a personnel manager at the Sale administration office. I was greeted by Philip's partner with the words 'What does it feel like to be the director of a failed company?'. Taken aback, I just smiled and thought to myself 'Are you an example of the way personnel management is conducted in this organisation?'. Then the next day, in a presentation to staff in Manchester, Allan Clarke stated that Independent was the only insurance company to have made a profit for all of the past five years. I knew that this was not true, because AIC had also posted five years of profit, but nevertheless I did not react immediately. That night in my hotel room I got copies of AIC's accounts and confronted Alan the next day with some facts. Alan was clearly unable to answer them, but dismissed it by saying to wait and see how the old AIC ran off.

I also soon learned that the accounting principles adopted by Independent were less conservative than those at AIC. Michael Bright had always been in sales and never directly involved in the risk-taking decisions of underwriting. The most important driving force to him was selling and premium income growth. At the same time, acquisition costs (not just commission paid to brokers but also the salary costs of staff engaged in business development, including mine) were being treated as deferred expenses in the balance sheet. This was fine while there was growth in premium income, but I knew that one day this would catch up and if it did then the likelihood was that the company would post losses and possibly become insolvent. The danger of having a sales-driven person at the helm of a financial services company has been proven since when Northern Rock Building Society ran into difficulty from expanding too fast into doubtful lending.

I could go on, but I think I have made my point and I do not want to lose my reader's interest.

Suffice it to say that it turned out that the Financial Services Authority, which regulated the insurance industry, were not used to dealing with a solvent company in run off. Most insurance companies went into run off because they were under-reserved—the FSA realised that AIC had been conservatively over-reserved. Within two years the FSA had authorised a £2 million dividend for AIC to pay to Holland. This had previously been unheard of, and several more dividends were subsequently authorised. In 2003, AIC was finally put into a Members Voluntary Liquidation, by which time a surplus of over £80 million had been repatriated to Holland by way of dividends and capital.

So much for the 'failed insurance company' that I had been a director of.

By contrast, in 2001 the non-executive directors of Independent spectacularly sacked Michael Bright; the company was placed in the hands of administrators and subsequently went into insolvent liquidation. Michael Bright, Philip Condon and Dennis Lomas were later convicted of fraud and each given custodial sentences.

In September 1996 I took my pay-off from Independent and left this period of my life behind me. Even this was a struggle. I had to fight to get my agreed severance terms. What annoyed me even more was that, as director of AIC responsible for staff, I was privy to confidential information relating to the transfer of pension rights to Independent. I knew that my own pension rights in 1994 were valued at £320,000 and when I left Independent I was offered an actuarially valued transfer-out value of £280,000. So much for actuaries! I challenged this and was offered a transfer amount of £380,000 so long as I did not pursue the matter. It still took until February 1997 for me to receive the payment in my personal pension plan.

Now, unemployed for the first time in my life, I was again faced with the inevitable question: WHAT WOULD YOU LIKE TO DO? What I really wanted to do was to turn the clock back to August 1994 and persuade the Dutch to refuse the Independent offer to acquire the AIC business to give us more time to agree a management buy-out.

John F. Kennedy once said:

> The one unchangeable certainty is that nothing is unchangeable or certain.

He was not wholly correct because what has happened **is** certain and **is not** changeable.

## Chapter 11
# PETER'S TIME

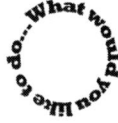

Jim Rohn (September 17 1930–December 5 2009) was an American entrepreneur, author and motivational speaker. He said once:

> Time is more valuable than money. You can get more money but you can't get more time.

I will attempt to explain my view of time. It is based on theories and facts, many of which are featured in Stephen Hawking's books and many of which can be neither proved nor disproved.

I have nothing but admiration for Stephen Hawking and have read some of his books, albeit with varying degrees of comprehension of physics and quantum theories. He is a truly remarkable man and I am fascinated by his theories of what time is in the context of our life and my belief.

Stephen Hawking is severely disabled by a motorneurone disease known as amyotrophic lateral sclerosis (ALS). Hawking's illness is markedly different from typical ALS in that his form of ALS is the most protracted case ever documented. A survival for more than ten years after diagnosis is uncommon for ALS; the longest documented durations are 32 and 39 years and these cases were termed benign because they lacked the typical progressive course. Stephen has survived for more than 47 years since diagnosis of his crippling illness.

Despite the apparent 'miracle' of his survival for so long with his illness, Stephen does not believe in God. Throughout his early work, Hawking used the word 'God' metaphorically but also suggests that the existence of God is unnecessary to explain the origin of the universe, as discussed in *A Brief History of Time*, and he does not believe in a personal God. He says:

The question is: 'is the way the universe began chosen by God for reasons we can't understand, or was it determined by a law of science'? I believe the second. Because there is a law such as gravity, the Universe can and will create itself from nothing.

His most recent book, The *Grand Design*, starts by saying:

We each exist for but a short time, and in that time explore but a small part of the whole universe. But humans are a curious species. We wonder, we seek answers. Living in this vast world that is by turns kind and cruel, and gazing at the immense heavens above, people have always asked a multitude of questions: How can we understand the world in which we find ourselves? How does the universe behave? What is the nature of reality? Where did all this come from? Did the universe need a creator? Most of us do not spend time worrying about these questions, but almost all of us worry about them some of the time.

Despite his belief that science can provide the answer to everything and therefore there is no need for a 'God' to explain the universe, nowhere in his book does he actually say or provide any evidence to suggest that God does not exist.

In the final part of his book he says:

The universe has a design, and so does a book. But unlike the universe, a book does not appear spontaneously from nothing. A book requires a creator.

Why does Stephen believe that 'the universe appears spontaneously from nothing'? His opinion is based on theories. By his own admission, theories are not laws of nature until such time as they are confirmed by incontrovertible observations. So why, until (if ever) these theories are proved to be laws of nature, cannot it be a possibility that the universe has a divine creator?

The most recent quantum theory that Stephen tries to explain is the M-theory. This theory accepts that time (or as the physicists call it 'space-time') is a dimension, not just one other dimension but 11 space-time dimensions. The M-theory also has solutions that allow perhaps as many as 10 to the power of 500 universes, each with its own laws! In Stephen's own explanation of this sort of magnitude of possibilities he states:

> If some being could analyse the laws predicted for each of those 10 to the power of 500 Universes in just one millisecond and had started working on it at the time of big bang, at present that being would have studied just 10 to the power of 20 of them. And that's without any coffee breaks.

Big bang happened over 13 billion years ago!

This may be the case, and Stephen may be able to deduce that the universe therefore appeared spontaneously from nothing, but to a layman such as me (and I suspect most of my readers) all this is less comprehensible than believing in God!

If everything can be explained by mathematics or rules of nature, how is randomness explained since, by definition, anything that is truly random cannot have any rule to govern it or, by definition, it would be predictable and therefore not truly random?

Like most subjects, mathematics has always fascinated me, and in particular the randomness of numbers or a series of numbers and particularly prime numbers (those that can only be divided by themselves or by 1, such as 1, 3, 5, 7, 11, 13, 17, 19).

It is a fascinating fact that prime numbers appear in a series which so far has been found to be totally random and cannot be predicted. Indeed, the systems of security which protect our credit cards, bank accounts and PINs can only function on the mathematics that uses prime numbers and the randomness and unpredictability in which they appear. If they are not truly random then it would be easy to break security codes.

And yet it is also a fact that every even number can be derived by adding two prime numbers together and every odd number can be derived from adding three prime numbers together. For example 16 can be derived from 11+5, 17 from 11+5+1, 18 from 13+5, 19 from 11+5+3, 20 from 13+7 or 17+3, and so on. Thus a law comes from a series that is truly random.

Another interesting series of numbers that a friend of mine showed me is as follows.

357,688,312,646,216,567,629,137
57,688,312,646,216,567,629,137
7,688,312,646,216,567,629,137
688,312,646,216,567,629,137
88,312,646,216,567,629,137
8,312,646,216,567,629,137
312,646,216,567,629,137
12,646,216,567,629,137
2,646,216,567,629,137
646,216,567,629,137
46,216,567,629,137
6,216,567,629,137
216,567,629,137
16,567,629,137
6,567,629,137
567,629,137
67,629,137
7,629,137
629,137
29,137
9,137
137
37
7

It is fascinating that each of these is a prime number and yet they form a pattern which is unpredictable—another illustration of order coming out of chaos.

I believe that only God, not laws of nature, can make order from randomness or chaos.

So, now, what is 'Peter's time'?

I can comprehend and believe that time is another dimension in addition to the three dimensions that we are able to experience every day in our three-dimensional world.

Imagine a world in which only two dimensions (length and width) can be perceived by its inhabitants; if the third dimension of depth (or height) is passed through this two-dimensional world, all that its inhabitants are able to perceive is an infinite number of different two-dimensional images.

We live in and are able to comprehend a three-dimensional world. If time, as another dimension, were passed through us we would only be capable of experiencing it as an infinite different number of three-dimensional images.

Whether or not you believe in miracles, everyone must accept (and many will have actually experienced) unexplained phenomena such as telepathy. The one thing that makes miracles and other phenomena unique is that they transcend time. An easy example is when Jesus turned water into wine. This is not an impossible thing for us mere mortal men to achieve, since the ingredients of wine are water, grapes, yeast and, of course, time. The miracle was that Jesus transcended time. The numerous occasions when Jesus healed the sick were only miracles because he did so instantly, again transcending time. We know that sick people can get better, given treatment and time.

There are other ways in which miracles happen when time is transcended. Perhaps Stephen Hawing, by living such a long life against all odds, is himself a beneficiary of a miracle.

William Cowper, in one of the *Twenty-Six Letters on Religious Subjects*, published by John Newton in 1774, wrote:

God moves in a mysterious way his wonders to perform.

It is reportedly the last hymn Cowper ever wrote, with a fascinating (though unsubstantiated) story behind it. Cowper often struggled with depression and doubt. One night he decided to commit suicide by drowning himself. He called a cab and told the driver to take him to the Thames river. However, thick fog came down and prevented them from finding the river (another version of the story has the driver getting lost deliberately). After driving around lost for a while, the cabby finally stopped and let Cowper out. To Cowper's surprise, he found himself on his own doorstep; God had sent the fog to keep him from killing himself. Even in our blackest moments, God watches over us.

I believe that God and his son in the form of Christ exist in a place that transcends time. I also believe that when we die we will move into a place in which time is constantly there as a new dimension and in which we too will exist alongside our Maker.

Albert Einstein, who is perhaps the father of modern theoretical physics, once said:

People like us, who believe in physics, know that the distinction between past, present and future is only a stubbornly persistent illusion.

# Chapter 12
# DOWNS AND UPS

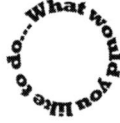

*...What would you like to do...*

Life is full of ups and downs. The trick is to enjoy the ups and
have courage during the downs. (Anon.)

At the end of 1993, Penny was just finishing her year as head
girl in Karen Dixon's yard when a horse reared up and landed on
her, crushing her pelvis and breaking it in four places. Duncan and I
went up to North Yorkshire and Duncan drove Penny's horse back
in the horsebox while I carefully took Penny home, in a lot of pain
and cushioned by pillows on the front seat of my car. She spent two
weeks in hospital without any operation and was told that she would
not ride competitively for the next 12 months. As usual, Penny did
not accept this and was back on a horse by the end of January 1994,
sitting on pillows across the saddle. She was competing again in
April.

As I have explained, The Terrace House where we lived had
been a great party house and had a two-acre garden. There were no
facilities for keeping horses. It was far too big and costly to maintain,
especially bearing in mind my situation with Independent and the
fact that my two-year contract would be over in September 1996.
At the end of 1994 Duncan, having lost jobs in the City, had signed
on for 12 months' service and was away training and then on a tour
in Northern Ireland. Penny wanted to start her own yard and build
a business teaching and training horses, so we started looking at a
move of house.

It took us until the beginning of 1995 to find our new home
at Lower Stunts Green Farm near Herstmonceux and complete sale
of The Terrace House. At the end of March 1995 we moved into
the farm, which is a charming property, parts of it dating back to
the 1600s and having 11 acres of fields and woodland, eight stables
and a large barn and five bedrooms. I was also able to reduce my
mortgage considerably, easing further the future strain on income.

So this was the first DOWN—a down-size in property, which did not require courage and was actually very enjoyable. The only negative was that it was a further and longer journey for me to travel to London. But I was prepared to accept this for the benefits that the move gave us. We spent ten very happy years at the farm until Alli's death. Penny and her husband John still live there.

In April 1995, Duncan had completed his training for deployment in Northern Ireland and had a few days' leave. Without telling us he decided to 'come home'. He drove to The Terrace House in Colemans Hatch, only to find that there were new owners and we had moved to Stunts Green. He did not know where this was, or our new telephone number. He went to the local pub and asked there and was given our telephone number. Poor neglected son—what horrible parents we must have been! When he phoned I told him we had set him an initiative test, and gave him directions to our new home.

In order to assist Penny we had a large outdoor school with an all-weather surface built and I built four additional stables. Penny started her own business and Alli and I helped by accommodating young trainee staff and looking after them. Alli always enjoyed 'adopting youngsters' and gave them a lot of grief when they did not keep their bedrooms tidy, but otherwise became a surrogate mum to them.

Duncan returned at the end of 1995 and we noticed a big change in him. We had not realised it, but he had been posted to East Tyrone with the Irish Guards. He has never fully disclosed to me what this involved, but I understand that he had some unpleasant tasks, and as a result of these experiences he had matured in a way that is difficult to describe. He had been sponsored by the Irish Guards to go on a regular commissioning board for possible admission to the Royal Academy Sandhurst (RMAS). He was not sure that this was what he wanted to do, but decided to go to Westbury on 2nd January 1996. He was philosophical about the possibility of failing, but said that if he did not try he would probably spend the rest of his life regretting it and wondering whether he should have done it. He returned home on 5th January not knowing whether he had passed, and at four o'clock that afternoon received a phone call telling him had passed and that there was a vacancy for him if he reported to RMAS no later than 1500 hours on Sunday 7th January. To be eligible for a commission in one of the front-line regiments, Duncan was on the border age-wise for entry to RMAS, so he had less than 48 hours to sort his life out and report.

Alli and I were very proud parents when we delivered Duncan to Sandhurst that Sunday afternoon and wished him well in his year as an officer cadet. We did not see or hear anything from him for the first six weeks of what he called 'bull and beasting', during which some of his colleagues on the intake walked out because they were not prepared to be treated that way. We were invited to a Sunday church parade and lunch at the end of his first six weeks. He was obviously enjoying his new life and was very proud to be treading the York stone corridors of Old College where so many great people, such as Sir Winston Churchill, had been before him. For the past 12 months, Duncan had been dating Sam Warburton, whom we had known for some years because she, Penny and Duncan had been in the Pony Club together. A lot of the leave that Duncan had he spent with Sam at her parents' home in the Ashdown Forest, so we did not see a great deal of him in 1996.

Alli and I settled into the new community and got involved in local village social life, which centred mainly on The Merry Harriers pub in Cowbeech, and made a lot of new friends. The Merry Harriers had a bonfire society and held functions to raise money to pay for Bonfire Night and give money to local charities and good causes. We joined the committee and spent five very happy years involved in this until Alli's health started to fail as her heart condition deteriorated. In particular, Dave and Mary Ann Gordon became great friends and are still to this day.

In September 1996 my contract with Independent expired and I was faced not so much with WHAT WOULD YOU LIKE TO DO? as WHAT CAN I DO? As many others who face redundancy or the end of an era of their career in their mid-fifties will know, it is not easy to find a new job at the level of seniority or income previously enjoyed. I was convinced that I could somehow find or create new opportunities and decided not to seek or apply for jobs advertised or contact agencies. I had attended a course with the Chartered Institute of Arbitrators and qualified as an associate member then joined the Academy of Experts, completing their excellent training course in being an expert witness in litigation, using my 'expertise' as an insurance underwriter, and put my details on the register of expert witnesses. I sent a mail shot to over 100 solicitors who I knew specialised in insurance litigation. Without any experience of being an expert witness under my belt, and no track record for recommendation in the legal profession, I had to sit and wait for opportunities to arise. I realised that I could not rely on expert witness work for any regular income and had to seek other opportunities. I went regularly to London and trudged the streets and bars making contact with colleagues with whom I had worked and other underwriters and brokers.

I met Richard King who had been the CEO of an Australian-owned London reinsurance company with which I had done business in the past. He was now a director of a small consultancy company called Richards & Pearson Limited (R&P) in Leadenhall Street. Richard had some great ideas about setting up new agencies and underwriting operations. This gave me a City base, and Richard and I brainstormed his ideas, one of which was to set up a new Friendly Society to provide insurance cover at a very cheap premium for personal accident compensation if policyholders were ever a victim of violent crime. I thought that this was an excellent idea, since the government scheme through the Criminal Injuries Compensation Board was a slow and painful process whereas, as a Friendly Society, we would be able to provide a fast and efficient claims service. I spent two years working on this and getting approval from the Friendly Societies Commission, with the financial backing of reinsurers. Somewhat naively, and without previous experience of marketing, I believed that we had developed a new product which would sell—but it did not, and the new society ran out of funds, which were mainly absorbed by R&P in administration costs. I took a minimal salary for only six months before resigning in the wake of heavy criticism for not having achieved budgeted sales targets.

Another DOWN, as I had put a lot of time and effort into a business venture that was not to succeed.

By contrast, at the same time came an UP.

When walking down Fenchurch Street in April 1997 I bumped into Allan Norton who had been a marine underwriter at AIC and, like the other AEGON staff, had been transferred to Independent. I asked Allan how things were going and he said:

> 'You obviously have not heard; three weeks ago Michael Bright gave me five minutes to clear my desk and leave and I am now looking for a new job and going for interviews'.

With not too much difficulty, I persuaded Allan to join me for a pint in The Elephant in Fenchurch Street and, knowing that Allan had good underwriting expertise in insuring yachts—particularly the really big superyachts that the very rich owned—over lunch I asked him if he would be interested in setting up his own underwriting agency. His response was that he had a big mortgage, his wife was about to have their first baby, he had no capital or management experience to know how to go about it. Although I had eaten into my cash reserves, I still had capital available to invest in a new venture. I also had the experience of management at senior level and R&P had the administration to support a new start-up underwriting agency. I introduced Allan to Richard King and, while Allan was still trying to seek a new job, we worked on setting up a new underwriting agency and attracting reinsurance support and a consortium of underwriters to back us. Richard's contacts and skills in selling a business plan and concept were invaluable, and in less than three months we set up Lead Yacht Underwriters Limited with a market-leading capacity of US$50 million for any one risk to underwrite superyachts. I personally put up all the capital and funded the cashflow and expenses in the early years.

In any new business achieving business plan targets is not easy. Business was slow because we were seen as the 'new boys' in the market among the established underwriters in this class (especially as we had much larger capacity than them) and Independent were very aggressive, undercutting premium rates through their closed broker network. For the first two and a half years we struggled to write sufficient business to cover our expenses, a period during which both Allan and I made sacrifices. Allan took a salary which was less that he could have earned elsewhere, and I took no salary. At the end of 1998 Vladimir Mirosecic Sorgo, a marine broker who in 1997 had helped us to put together the consortium of underwriting backers for Lead Yacht, was made redundant. Very bravely, as Vlad had a young family and a mortgage, he decided to take a sabbatical and study for an MBS at the City of London University. Allan invited Vlad to be a non-executive director of Lead Yacht and, to help him, the company sponsored Vlad to write a thesis as part of his studies on the superyacht industry.

As I said, the support that R&P gave us in 1997 was invaluable in helping us set up Lead Yacht. The managing director and main shareholder of R&P was a lady called Janet Pearson who was a chartered accountant. Allan and I were both concerned that Janet, like many ladies in management I have met, was a bit of a 'control freak', and by 1999 Allan was at the end of his tether, with Janet trying to interfere in the way the company was being run. With income below plan, R&P were also draining the company's revenue and cashflow with administration charges. In May 1999 Allan came to see me at home and said that, unless we could extract ourselves from R&P and go it alone, he would resign and seek other opportunities. As anyone who has been involved in business partnerships knows, that extraction can be a very painful process, especially if there are any loose ends in contractual arrangements. Luckily, when we set up Lead Yacht I engaged the services of a long-time family friend, Tim Wells. Apart from being a personal friend, Tim was the commercial partner of Pannone and Partners, solicitors based in Manchester. Tim and I had worked together in the past when he had helped me personally and advised AIC in some of its trade investments, particularly in the painful exercise of putting P S Mosse & Partners into liquidation in 1993. Tim had done a thorough job when we set up Lead Yacht in 1997 in drafting watertight contracts and a shareholders agreement. I again asked Tim to help us to extricate Lead Yacht from R&P. Initially I made an offer to purchase the shares that R&P owned, but was told by Janet Pearson that the company was 'worth nothing'. Janet was not happy about losing control over Lead Yacht but, having agreed to honour the service contract fees, we held a Board meeting at which the deal was done and Janet was asked to resign as company secretary, which she did with some reluctance. Her parting words as she left the board meeting were:

> 'Gentlemen, I would like to say it was a pleasure to do business with you but it was not'.

Ten minutes later Vlad received a telephone call from Janet, who said to him that her parting words were not meant for him. We have since constantly reminded Vlad that obviously Janet did not consider him to be a gentleman. This is the same Janet who objected to my calling her female staff "ladies"!

We had two weeks to find new accommodation, and just before Christmas 1999 we moved into a temporary office, then early in January 2000 took a five-year lease on the offices which were to remain the home of Lead Yacht behind the 'glass gherkin' in Bury Street. This meant that I had to provide the funds to pay off the R&P service charge and give my personal guarantee for the rent and to secure the company's bank overdraft to provide working capital. This meant that in 2000, had it gone wrong, I would have personally been in hock to the tune of more than £120,000. Vlad had finished his MBA degree and he now joined us as a working director, and we recruited a general assistant to carry out the administration. Luckily, Adam Wilson who was still with the AIC run off had Jeremy Ledger, a very capable assistant accountant, who was not fully occupied. Adam allowed us to use Jeremy to manage our accounts and set up systems to handle the business and payroll. The job grew as Lead Yacht expanded, and this arrangement worked out well for all parties, Jeremy joining us full-time in 2003 after AIC had wound up.

As I mentioned, from 1997 until only recently I acted as an underwriting expert witness in insurance litigation. I found this work both challenging and rewarding. The way that the English legal system operates in the High Courts is fascinating, and it is exciting to be part of it. In particular I have great admiration for barristers, who have an incredible intellect and a talent for reading briefs and instantly identifying the relevant points to be addressed. During the 14 years that I have been involved, I have given expert opinions on over 100 cases. Only a small percentage (fewer than 10%) ever go the whole way to trial. In the rest there is a settlement out of court or the action is withdrawn by one of the parties. I had the experience of cross-examination of my evidence and opinions as an expert on many occasions. While at times it is not a very pleasant experience, I have nothing but admiration for the way judges and barristers conduct trials, very politely and considerately. What you see as aggressive cross-examination in American films and television programmes is far from the reality of the English High Courts of Justice.

There are two, totally different, cases in which I have been involved which are worthy of mention.

The first followed the horrific terrorist attacks on the Twin Towers in New York, which I will not attempt to comment on except in so far as my involvement as an expert adviser to Silverstein Properties who owned the buildings was concerned. Silverstein purchased the Twin Towers from the Port Authority of New York in early 2001, less than nine months before the attack. It was agreed that the existing insurance policy would continue in force until June and then Silverstein would arrange their own insurance cover. At the time that the Towers were destroyed, although the insurance cover had been placed, the policy wording had not been agreed. The dispute was whether there were two separate losses, or only one loss arising from a single event (the terrorist attack). This was a fascinating case, in which I was asked for my opinion regarding London insurance market underwriting practice in the absence of an agreed wording.

The money at stake was in excess of £3 billion and I understand that eventually the dispute was settled out of court.

The other case, Pedley v Avon Insurance, was completely different. On 22 October 1993 the claimant, Derrick Pedley, suffered serious injuries from a fire which occurred while he was carrying out work to a BMW at the motor car premises where he was employed. The case was not heard until ten years later in 2003, so the memories of witnesses were a bit cloudy. The motor repair business was owned by a Mrs Moody, and the main issue in the case was whether or not she failed to disclose to her insurers the fact that her husband, Mr Roy Moody, an undischarged bankrupt, was a person connected with the ownership or management of the business. I was asked as an expert underwriting witness to give my opinion, particularly relating to this issue. In his summing up, the judge referred to part of my evidence and said:

> I do not consider that, in the light of my findings, Avon has been able to pass the Sangster test (if I may so describe it) set out at paragraph 3.1 of his report. I conclude, therefore, that Avon has not shown that Mrs Moody's answer to question 6.3 on the proposal form was incorrect, or that she was therefore responsible for a material misrepresentation or non-disclosure or for a breach of warranty under the basis clause.

This was an UP.

The Sangster test may never be used or referred to again, but I am responsible for a precedent in English Law which will stand for ever.

Duncan had passed out of Sandhurst in December 1996 and been awarded a regular commission in the 22nd (Cheshire) Regiment. It was two very proud parents who attended the parade and, although it was a bit wet and cold, I still have fond memories of the day.

One of our UPs!

By 2001 Duncan was Adjutant of the Cheshires and stationed in Cyprus. Alli and I decided we would have a holiday in Northern Cyprus in September, hoping that Duncan would be able to get a pass to visit us some time during the holiday. We had not realised how difficult this would be, or the strong antagonism and dislike the Greek Cypriots had for the Turkish and vice versa. Duncan was not sure that he would be able to get a pass but said he would try. After four days, Alli's ankles started to swell, she did not feel well and was short of breath; when the local doctor visited her, he immediately took her to a small private hospital in Famagusta where a specialist said that she was suffering from a heart condition and kept her in for a week. The small hospital was very comfortable, but right opposite was a large mosque and so Alli enjoyed the delight of the call to prayers five times a day. By the time she returned to the apartment Duncan had managed to get not just a pass but a blue-light escort to the border, so he came to visit us. Alli had been put on heart medication and told to go and see her doctor as soon as we returned to the UK.

On return, Alli's doctor immediately referred her to a heart specialist in Eastbourne Hospital and she spent the next four weeks in intensive care suffering from fibrillation and heart failure. The specialist said that her heart was badly diseased and the only cure would be a transplant. I asked for her to be put on the list for a transplant but the specialist advised that it was highly unlikely that she would get one because any match would first be offered to a younger patient and she, being 57, would be at the bottom of the priority list.

This was a real DOWN.

Alli was given a course of Warfarin and other heart medication and it was not until February 2002 that the specialist defibrillated her heart which then, as much as it could, returned to normal. However, from then until her death in November 2003 she was not able to return to her normal active self and to all intents and purposes was an invalid.

In the meantime, Lead Yacht was developing at a steady rate. Because Vlad was working full-time Allan could spend more of his energies networking and increasing the company's profile, and I was able to share the work involved with accounting and financial business planning so that I could devote more time to Alli. At Lead Yacht we had a non-executive director on the Board representing our leading consortium underwriting. In early 2002 I was concerned that such a non-executive director would not be totally impartial, and proposed that we seek a director who would be totally independent and who could bring missing expertise and advise us on corporate matters from a fresh point of view. It is also in accordance with best recommended corporate practice to have independent directors to advise on such matters as directors' remuneration and internal auditing. I suggested asking Andy Ripley, whom I had known as a friend for some years. Vlad was not immediately convinced, so I asked

Andy if he might consider it and, if so, to come and meet us. At the meeting, Vlad's concerns were dispelled when he realised that Andy had been a Name at Lloyd's for some years, and was a chartered accountant with degrees in economics and business studies. Andy said that he would be happy to join the board so long as we were not asking him to do so because of 'his blond hair and big tits'! (referring to his celebrity status as a rugby player). The word 'great' is the best to describe Andy. Apart from the fact that whenever he approved or agreed with something he would say 'that's great', he was a great man and a great help to us all, and the encouragement and love which he grew to have for Lead Yacht over the next eight years until his death from prostate cancer in 2010 were an inspiration to us all. We all miss Andy and his great sense of humour and enthusiasm.

By 2006, Lead Yacht had grown to an extent that I was being paid a salary and Allan and Vlad were starting to be stretched. In order to continue growing we clearly needed another good underwriter. We approached Iain Cotton, who had been a marine underwriter and had supported Lead Yacht but was now working as a broker and wanted to get back into underwriting. Iain was pleased to be asked, and joined us as another director and shareholder. Iain's arrival heralded a three-year period of further growth and profitability for Lead Yacht.

When Andy was diagnosed with prostate cancer in 2007 he wrote to me and said he would quite understand if we wished him to step down because of the treatment he would have to undergo and the future uncertainties. I wrote a reply saying:

> 'You will have to come up with a better excuse than that, Andy'.

2007 was also Lead Yacht's tenth anniversary year, so in October we held a celebratory dinner for brokers, yacht captains and yacht brokers at the Cavalry and Guards Club at which we held an auction in aid of the Prostate Cancer Charity and raised over £16,000. Chris Noe, our claims manager, kept a pair of slippers in the office in which he rested his feet and, unknown to Chris, Vlad had nicked them as one of the auction items. They fetched £250, bid by a solicitor who knew Chris well—but I wonder how well! I think they were returned to Chris afterwards.

Seeing Lead Yacht grow and succeed while having great fun at work was another wonderful UP.

During this time, Penny was developing her equestrian business and competing in the UK, Ireland and France. At one event she represented England. Alli and I were very proud. Although Penny did not (and still does not particularly) like teaching, it is an essential part of her income to enable her to continue eventing horses, which is her real passion. We would frequently go to support her when we could, but I was always terrified by the size of some of the cross-country jumps. They were so solid that if you were to hit one of them there was a real chance that the horse would somersault and a real risk of serious injury to the rider. Very little protective clothing will save you from a ton of horse landing on you, and eventing as a sport has more fatalities that most others, including motor car racing which, because of technology, is now a relatively safe sport.

For those who do not know much about eventing except watching Badminton on television, there are three elements. The first, after the horses have been vetted to make sure they are sound, is the dressage, where the horse and rider have to show discipline in complex riding movements. The second day is the endurance phase. The rules were changed in 2006, but before that it was not just cross-country jumping. First there were up to 24 kilometers of roads and tracks which the horse had to complete at a working trot, followed by a four-kilometer steeplechase course to jump at a canter half-way, then the horse entered what is called a ten-minute box. The horse was checked again by a veterinary surgeon to make sure that it was still sound and the rider could check and change tack (most of the riders just chain-smoked and let their grooms do the work). In 1992, when Alli and I were watching Penny compete at Windsor, as she entered the ten-minute box another rider had a bad fall (which turned out to be a fatal accident) and she and other riders were kept waiting for over an hour while the air ambulance attended. Imagine, apart from losing the thrust of the adrenaline, the psychological effect on the riders of having to wait, knowing that something serious had happened. After the ten-minute box came the cross-country jumping. So if you have ever watched Badminton on television, remember what an endurance-testing phase this was. The next day again all the horses are vetted, and the show-jumping phase follows.

In 2006 I was watching Penny at Brightling. She was the first to go on the cross-country and I was beside the water complex and could see her approach the third jump, where the horse decided to put its front feet down in between a spread fence. The inevitable happened. I saw Penny somersault through the air, closely followed by the horse, also somersaulting. My heart went into my mouth and I ran as fast as I could across the fields. Fortunately she suffered nothing worse than a broken arm.

A DOWN and an UP within minutes of each other!

I explain all this because I am so proud of Penny and her achievements in a sport which demands great skill and courage.

In October 2003, Alli and I went to Italy on holiday for a week with John and Anne, Alli's cousin and his wife. Towards the end Alli was not feeling too good, and was very tired but not showing any of the signs of the problems she had had in Northern Cyprus two years earlier. When we got home, I tried to persuade Alli to go and see our doctor but she refused, saying that she was all right. I now wish that I had been more persuasive.

Less than three weeks later Alli died.

It was a Friday evening and I had taken the dogs for a walk at about nine o'clock. I was in the kitchen and heard a bang and immediately went into the lounge to find Alli collapsed and not breathing. I immediately phoned 999 and started resuscitation procedures as best I knew them. It took the ambulance nearly half an hour to arrive—the worst 30 minutes of my life. By this time Penny had arrived, and the paramedics were trying to resuscitate Alli, to no avail. Penny kindly agreed to follow the ambulance to the hospital as I felt too exhausted and was expecting Duncan to arrive any moment. Alli was pronounced dead on arrival Eastbourne General Hospital.

The biggest DOWN I have ever suffered.

As befitted a wonderful and loving lady, Alli's funeral was attended by many friends and relatives who had travelled great distances. The cortège was led by a mounted escort with James, Lucy, Lauren, Carly, Natalie and Tish riding, all of them students who had worked for Penny and whom Alli and I had looked after, living as part of the family. As the cortège drove through Herstmonceux to the church, all the shopkeepers came out and paid tribute. It was all very moving and emotional. For the service I chose that *The Lord is my Shepherd* be sung to the tune written by Howard Goodall for the Vicar of Dibley theme; I know Alli would appreciate that.

During the last year of her life, Alli wrote a number of poems about her life experiences and people and animals. After her death I had these made into a book called *Alli's Poems* and in memory of Alli I have attached it as an appendix to this book.

We had three dogs at the time: Spanner, a springer spaniel, Tara a black labrador and Caly, a newfoundland. At the end of November, two weeks after Alli's funeral, I first went back to the office in London. It was a wet, cold November day and Penny phoned me when I was on the train coming home to say that Tara and Caly had run off and she did not know where they were. When I arrived home, they had been found two miles from the house, both killed by a lorry or some other passing vehicle on the road.

Another DOWN.

I said to Penny that they were probably looking for Alli and had now found her. Spanner has since been my closest friend, and he follows me everywhere, not wanting to leave me.

After Alli's death, my world was lonely and I was living in an empty space. I tried to get on with life but Christmas with Penny and Duncan was a sad event. Duncan returned to his duties in the Army. Early in January 2004 I rented a villa in Antigua and took Penny for a two-week holiday. This turned out to be a great relief for both of us. We had a wonderful time and it helped us to try and look forward instead of backwards. However, on return to 'normal' life I started to drift downwards into a deep pit, with a feeling of self-guilt and drinking and smoking far too much. I have since been told that this is quite a normal reaction to a traumatic event such as bereavement. I was also suffering badly from a pain in my right elbow, and a consultation with my orthopedic surgeon confirmed that my rheumatoid arthritis had caused the joint to all but completely disintegrate and it was in need of replacement.

Not so much a question of WHAT WOULD YOU LIKE TO DO? as of WHAT ARE YOU GOING TO DO?

Our old friends Sue and Tim Wells were going to the Algarve for a week's holiday at the beginning of March and asked me to join them. This I did, and because Sue and Tim played a fair amount of golf I had a lot of time to myself to do some serious heart-searching and thinking. I decided that I had to pull myself together and get on with life. The first thing was to have the elbow replacement operation, which I arranged immediately after my return. The pain disappeared overnight. This was such a relief that only then did I realise that I had been in constant pain 24/7 for over a year. The second thing that I decided was that I am not the sort of person who can cope on my own and that I need personal companionship and love. How do I go about finding another partner who could in any way replace Alli?

The practicalities of how to go about meeting new people—in a pub, join a Bridge club or wander the streets with a notice around my neck? I had heard of the then relatively new website called Friends Reunited and I decided on my return to try and see if I could make contact with old school and teenage friends to see whether I could find some re-acquaintances after all these years.

I Googled 'friends' and one of the first sites that appeared was one called Make Friends on Line. I studied this and decided that it was a secure way in which I could find new friends in the comfort of my own home and without the hassle of personal contact unless I wished to. I enrolled and put some information about myself on-line using the code name LYUL. Over the next few weeks I got great comfort from chatting electronically with some lovely ladies, not just in the UK but also in Florida, British Columbia, the Caribbean and New Jersey, each with her own lonely story. I met one lady who lived in Reigate a few times and we got on very well, but it was only ever going to be a friendship and we agreed there was no mileage in trying to pursue a relationship. Then one evening a lady codenamed LCC who lived in Bexhill-on-Sea contacted me. I said to her that I would be on-line all evening if she wanted a chat; then by accident I must have clicked the Block Contact button. I heard no more from LCC and thought she had decided that she had no interest in me, so I forgot about this contact. Unknown to me, LCC had tried several times to contact me over the next week. I subsequently learned that LCC did not know why she persisted in trying as I was really not 'her cup of tea', but after a week she contacted the website to ask whether there was a reason why I had not responded to her. The website sent me an email pointing out that I had blocked LCC and asked if I had intended to. I told them that I had not, and they unblocked LCC and we started to chat, eventually meeting for coffee one Saturday morning in early May at a café in Battle.

The second I walked into the café and set my eyes on Linda I felt that chemistry which is impossible to explain. Within two weeks, Linda came to Portugal with me for a week's holiday, and on the ferry from Portsmouth to Bilbao I proposed to Linda just 13 days after we had met; foolishly she said YES. I now believe that all this was what I can only describe as divine providence.

This was an UP; most of the rest, as they say, is history!

During the past ten years I have become involved in charitable work. In 2002 I was approached by John Manley, who was then the chief executive officer of Sussex Archaeological Society (SAS), who asked if I would consider becoming a co-opted member of the finance and administration committee (F&A). I had no real interest in history or archaeology and was fascinated to learn that SAS had more than 2000 members and owned nine properties in Sussex including Michelham Priory, Fishbourne Roman Palace and Lewes Castle, and had a budget of £1.5 million. At the time the SAS was looking to co-opt on to F&A someone with a business background and the skills that were lacking among the trustees. My name had been given to John by our next-door neighbour, Frizzie, who worked at Michelham Priory. I agreed, and this was the start of nine years' association with the SAS during which time I was elected a trustee, chaired F&A and for the last three years, until I retired in May 2011, was Chairman of the Council of Trustees.

In 2004, I was approached again, by a small charity called the Rural Community Support Society which runs the village Information Centre in Herstmonceux. The Centre was opened by the local churches as an outreach and community support in 1998, and I remember Alli at the time telling me what a wonderful project it was and how nice and helpful the volunteers were who staffed the Centre. The charity had run into financial problems and was holding an appeal and talking to the Parish Council to gain support. The Parish Council requested that the board of trustees be widened and that a proper business plan be prepared before it would consider financial support. I became a trustee and the treasurer and helped to secure grants from the Parish Council and other community grants and donations. In April 2011 I retired as a trustee, having secured for the Centre a deal where it has now purchased the freehold which secures its long-term future. I was able to dedicate this in Alli's memory. After meeting Linda, I began attending Beulah Baptist Church in Bexhill, which was a great source of Christian comfort and friendship. I spent two years as a deacon and for five years handled the Gift Aid system before retiring from these duties when I was first diagnosed in July 2010. I now have no mainstream charitable commitments, but I will continue to undertake charitable work as a way of putting back into society in general the experience and knowledge gained over my working years.

Linda had lost her husband, Tom, in April 2003. Apparently Tom was only 50 years old, fit and a non-smoker, who in January 2003 started with a husky throat which persisted. It was not until tests were taken in March 2003 that he was diagnosed with lung cancer which by then had already spread to secondary tumours. Sadly, Tom died in less than six months from his diagnosis. When I met Linda in May 2004, she owned a seafront flat in Bexhill which she wanted to sell so she could move, following Tom's death. After proposing to Linda, I suggested that we look for a house together in Bexhill. We found and bought 13 South Cliff Avenue, which is a delightful house with views over Pevensey Bay to Eastbourne and Beachy Head, and we spent the next three months having the house modernised and redecorated. Linda had to live through the chaos while I remained in Herstmonceux until January 2006 when, on my 61st birthday, Linda and I got married and we moved into our new home together. We are very happy in our home and at the time of writing are having a large extension built, so it is chaos and dust again, which this time we are sharing! I have to say that I am the luckiest man in the world because I can honestly say that I have been privileged to have the joy of the love and affection of the two most wonderful women in the world, Alli and Linda.

Linda has two sons, James and Ben. Needless to say they, as well as my own Penny and Duncan, were a little unsure when Linda and I first met, and had concerns about whether our relationship was 'the right thing'. There was never any friction or problems (except that Duncan and James did not seem to hit it off at first for some reason). I now treat and love James and Ben as if they were my own sons, and Linda feels the same about Penny and Duncan. In particular, Linda is no longer the wicked step-mother to Penny but just plain Mum. We are now as one family and, as I finish writing, Penny and her partner John Hill were married on 25th June 2011 and the party was at Lower Stunts Green Farm. Again, many old friends and family from afar travelled to help us celebrate the happy occasion. I was a very proud Dad and we had a great party.

All this is another big UP. What a lucky man I am.

From 2007 until 2010 Lead Yacht continued its steady and profitable growth. By 2010 the premium annual income written had risen to $35 million with substantial profits for the size of the company. The underwriting results were excellent, consistently providing an annual return on capital in excess of 50% for its underwriting backers. Over the previous three years we had had some talks with prospective companies which showed an interest in acquiring Lead Yacht but which had not resulted in any suitable offers. However, in

May 2010 within three weeks we received unsolicited approaches from three companies asking whether we were interested in selling Lead Yacht. I prepared an information memorandum and in July sent it to each of them, setting out the minimum deal that we would consider. In the middle of August one of the three, Amlin plc, an insurance company based in the Lloyd's market and quoted on the London Stock Exchange, agreed in principle and subject to due diligence and contract to acquire Lead Yacht at a price and terms which met our minimum requirements. It took from then until the beginning of 2011 to go through the process of due diligence and contractual negotiations to complete the deal, but in February 2011 Lead Yacht was sold to Amlin and I finally retired. I only wish that Andy Ripley had still been with us because I know he would have been very proud of what we had achieved in just 13 years of trading.

All this was another great UP.

A huge DOWN was in June 2010.

It was only a week after Andy's funeral and I was diagnosed with lung cancer and subsequently decided to write this book. I have now undergone chemotherapy and radiotherapy which has given the 'thing' a nasty fright, but it has not been eradicated. I am now on three-monthly scans and watch. I know that some time I will require further treatment but in the meantime I have been told to get on and enjoy life.

I am doing just that with the support of my fantastic and loving family and my many friends.

Kevin Welch in his song *Life Down Here on Earth* (1996) had a lyric which seems to me to be a great motto by which to go on living:

> There'll be two dates on your tombstone. And all your friends will read 'em. But all that's gonna matter is that little dash between 'em.

## Chapter 13
# WHERE NOW?

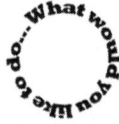

In the first chapter I reflected on the question WHAT WOULD YOU LIKE TO DO?

I hope that from reading my experiences you have thought about your own and life's trials and tribulations, especially those times of uncertainty or sadness caused by unexpected events.

I have included several times in my life when there were unexpected or unplanned events or changes outside my control. These often resulted, at best, in worrying about what would happen to me when my hopes had been dashed and I was faced with a future which I did not anticipate and, at worst, feeling that I was not able to cope with the future and suffering real low points.

My six cycles of chemotherapy caused me no serious side-effects, but an intense course of radiotherapy did. My radiotherapy treatment involved me driving from home to Maidstone. My appointments were early in the morning and from home the journey to Maidstone was a nightmare—all country roads, no dual carriageways or motorways. It took at least one and a half hours each way and the total time of each treatment was less than 15 minutes—a real bore! When I consider the impact that concentrated irradiation has on the body, it is not surprising that it made me feel very tired. It left me with a very irritating dry cough and my oesophagus was extremely sore so I had constant indigestion and discomfort. I was told that this was not unusual and that within a few weeks it would pass, which it did.

It is my nature to fight, but after radiotherapy, for the first time in my life I felt that I was no longer in control and could not fight what was happening to me.

This is yet another example of a situation when I was faced with the question WHAT WOULD YOU LIKE TO DO?

The best thing is to realise this and respond positively. Often not very easy!

Some of the other things my dear old Mum, in her unique way, used to say were:

'Every time a door closes another one slams in you face', and 'Every silver cloud has a bloody great big black lining around it'.

Comedy is often stating or twisting the obvious, and these are wonderful twists on how we tend conventionally to look at life. I am grateful that Mum's humour has helped me to cope with adversity on more than one occasion. Hers was a wonderful philosophy of life. In many troubled times when faced with adversity I have tried to be positive, pull myself together and look for new opportunities out of the debris instead of continuing to go further downhill by moping over what has happened.

And so my answer when, as we drove away from Conquest Hospital in June 2010, Linda asked me:

## WHAT WOULD YOU LIKE TO DO?
was:

'to spend whatever time I have left to do those things I can do which in a busy and sometimes selfish life I had neglected and had lost the realisation of their importance'.

These are:

First and foremost, to use all my strength and will power to fight my illness and prove the medical profession wrong, not in their diagnosis, which I accept, but in their prognosis.

Second, to enjoy to the absolute full the love, friendship, strength and support of my wonderful family and many friends.

Third, to try and use all my natural senses more and fill myself with appreciation of all the wonderful things in everyday life—the weather, sunny, rainy or cold, the flora and fauna, and even man-made things of beauty and fascination.

Finally, to sort out all those things that I have ignored or 'put to one side'. I am the world's worst person at organising myself, and my filing and records are always left to the last minute to sort out. Now I may only have a last minute left, so the sooner I get on with this task the better!

You may notice that my answer to the question does not contain any material wishes.

Maybe this is just my nature, influenced by my life's experiences.

To explain this, although I have always enjoyed sports I have never been particularly good at any of them. I have learned that taking part always had to be the enjoyment. As far as I am concerned, the rare occasions of actually winning were the icing on the cake and not the reason for competing. The real pleasure has always been in taking part rather than the material rewards of winning. So to me material things, while often giving me immense pleasure and joy for a moment, have never really been as lastingly satisfying as being part of life itself.

As a tailpiece, you may have gathered that I have great pleasure in other people's quotations and thoughts on life. These often carry a lot of meaning and philosophy in a very few words, so I will end by quoting one of my best friends, Andy Ripley, one of many people who by his attitude and views on life had a strong influence on me. Andy, who died in June 2010 after a five-year brave fight against prostate cancer, wrote in his book:

> Dare we hope? We dare.
> Can we hope? We can.
> Should we hope? We must.
> We must, because to do otherwise is to waste the most precious of gifts, given so freely by God to all of us.
> So when we die, it will be with hope and it will be easy and our hearts will not be broken.

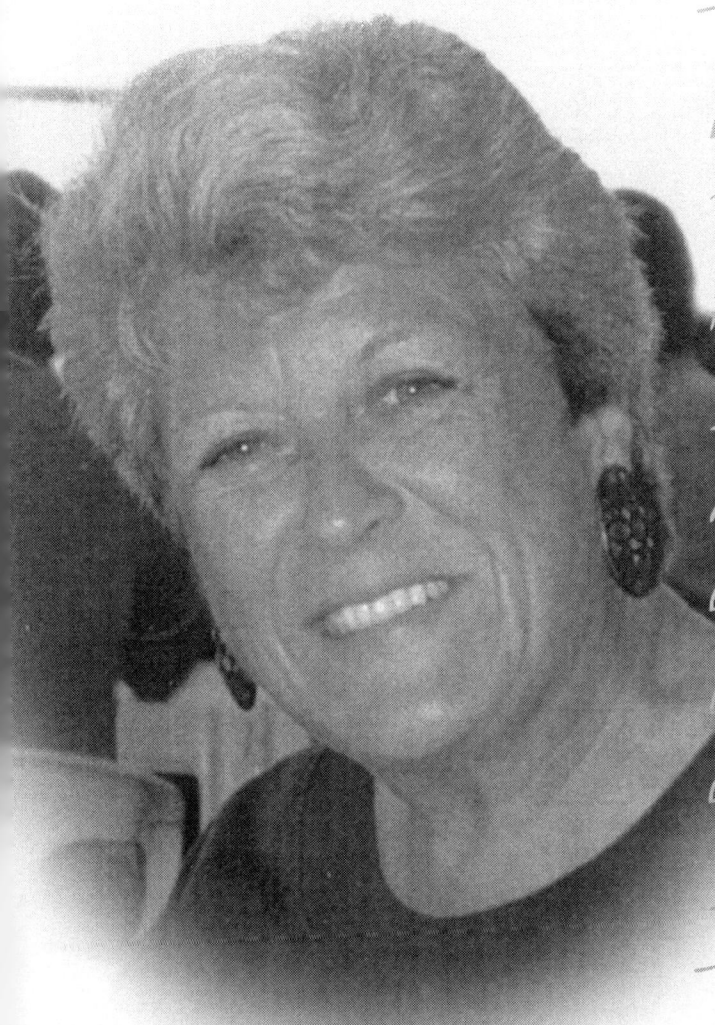

I've just cho

So I'll wri

They may r

But you'll t.

My Dad's g

For a year

I wish he w

P'raps he's g

When the h

Boy, do I sh

Will it just

I'll spoil t.

They should

Or at least

The neighbo

They don't

But soon I'l

# ALLI'S
# POEMS

# INTRODUCTION

In the last year of her life,
Alli, my darling wife,
Wrote poems from her heart -
A real talent and art;
It was her ambition and aim
To publish the same.

The characters in this book
Are just as true as they may look
And any likeness in appearances
Are based on Alli's life's experiences.
So I hope that you will grin and bear it
And if the cap fits, you will wear it!

This book contains those
Of her amusing prose
That she wrote with affection
For our recollection;
So it's dedicated by me
To her fond memory.

Peter.

# Alli's Apology

The magic pencil writes
And having written
It takes my breath away
But as a born Briton
I like the way words explode
Upon the virgin paper
The shape, the sound, the mode
What makes the words so clear,
Is, when spoken sound sincere.

There will become a time
When poetry and rhyme
Will go totally out of my head
And instead of a stanza
There'll be a bonanza –
Perhaps it was something that I said!

# A SPANNER IN THE WORKS

I've just changed homes
So I'll write some poems!
They may not rhyme
But you'll think they're fine
My Dad's gone away
For a year and a day
I wish he were here
P'raps he's gone for a beer!
When the humans go out
Boy, do I shout!
Well it just isn't done
I'll spoil their fun!
They should stay at home
Or at least leave me a bone
The neighbours will ring
They don't like that I sing
But soon I'll settle down
When I know where's my home!

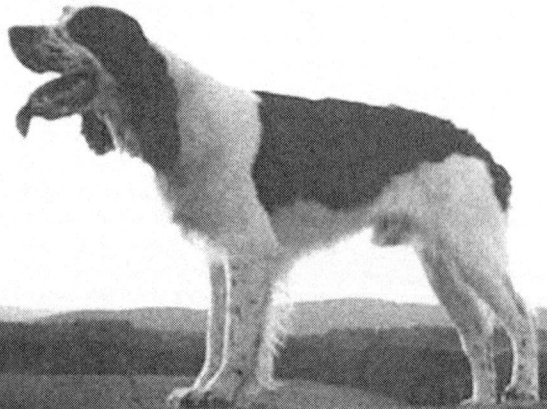

# AUNTY MARY

Aunty Mary's coming to tea
Tomorrow, Tuesday at half past three.
Cucumber sandwiches – they will be nice
And a real sponge cake, that I can help ice.
And those little buns with sugar and spice
I know they're her favourites – they're really nice

Uncle George will bring her – he always comes
He's a funny old soul, all fingers and thumbs.
Very carefully he'll settle her down on a chair
In her cask, where she lives – well she died last year.

# CHRISTOPHER BENJAMIN

Christopher Benjamin was a recruit
He joined on Monday in his best suit
On Tuesday he was off to war
By Wednesday he'd won by half past four
Thursday he started his second attack
By Friday he was getting the knack
On Saturday Russia was part of his aim
Sunday he'd really gone off this game
So that's what happens if you buy the disc
Of that time consuming Game called Risk!

# LITTLE WILLIE

Little Willie – sick in bed
Had a thought run through his head
"What if I could fly at night
Wouldn't that give Ma a fright?
She'd think I was a Vampire Bat
And not just me in a funny hat!"

Little Willie, feeling better
Wrote his Ma a lovely letter
Telling her about his dream
How he could fly, so it would seem
This brought his Ma to floods of tears
'Cos she had been a Witch for years.

Ma wrote back to Little Willie
Said "My dear, do not be silly
I know that you can fly at night
When stars are out and moon is bright.
It's time to fly on a broom stick
Now that you are no longer sick."

Little Willie, not a Ghoul
Was sent to learn at Hogwarts School
Of witchcraft, spells and other things
Like how to fly without wings.
'Twas there he met one Potter, Harry
And the girl he'd later marry.

The reason for this silly rhyme
Is, I dream too from time to time,
Of being famous, or a king
Tony Blair, J.K.Rowling.
If this could have ever been
Then I'd be richer than the Queen!

# Murphy

Now, Murphy, he was quite a lad
In fact, sometimes, was downright bad!
Issue he had in town and port
(And I do not mean the printed sort!)
He dressed to kill, and was a dandy
But beneath his jacket he was randy!
Chat-up lines he found a bore
That was not what his time was for!
He usually charged the same amount
And even opened his own "Bonk" account!
But the girls, they fell for this obvious cad
And many were heard to say "Hello, Dad"
So next time you see a bitch with a grin,
Lorry Park Lad's been at it again!

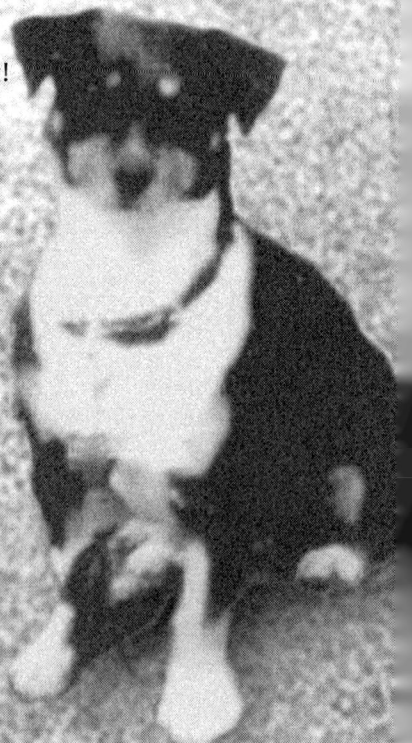

# MY BEST FRIEND

My best friend – I'll call her Mable
Said "Please don't clear the coffee table"
There's things I haven't seen for years
Wait, I'll start and stem your fears.

There's magazines and catalogues
And fluffy bits off the dogs
A pair of socks – oh, not a pair!
A golf ball and some underwear
A lace up shoe,
Some super glue
A brown and furry kangaroo
A used tea plate
An after eight
A ticket for the London Tate
A blue band-aid
Some lemonade
And half a jar of marmalade
A piece of cheese
A cat with fleas
A melted pack of frozen peas
A piece of toast
Some Sunday roast
A post card from the Irish Coast
A where am I?
A well dead fly
A photo from the London Eye
A pink rosette
A brown hair net
A duster and a serviette
A cigarette
A cruet set
My favourite sort of vinaigrette
Some indian ink
A bow that's pink
The contents of the kitchen sink
A book by who?
A How-do-you-do
A what's-it-called,
And there are two!
A juicy orange,
And a.......
        zzzz....

        zzzzzz.......

        ZZZZZZZZZZZZZZZZ....................

# OAP's

Forget the gin and tonic
Think more of tonic wine
The pair of glasses on the chair –
Are they yours or mine?

Elastic stockings, Sterodent
Senatogen and pills
Are scattered round the bedroom
To sort out little ills.

There's not a lot to recommend
The fact we're growing older
With creaky joints and rotten teeth
And nasty, stiff cold shoulder

But one thing that can make us smile
Is the "Pimpley's" grow old too
They're becoming "Wrinkleys"
And we "Crumbley's" say "Yah Sucks Boo"!

# PEARS

Oh how I remember
That day in September
When I saw that tree full of pears
I picked and I ate
And I'll not forget
How I blew myself right up stairs!

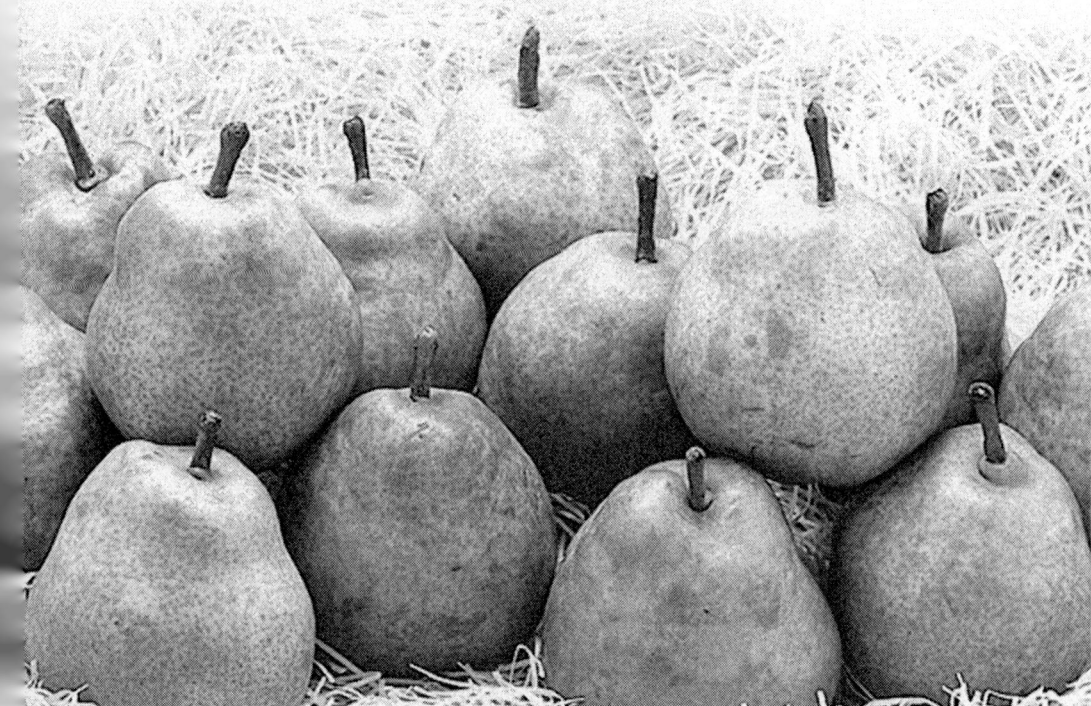

Oh, it is so nice
Kindly pass the ice
Oh, it is so hot
I'm a big grease spot
Oh, I need a drink
One that's pretty pink
Oh, I need a drink
Filled up to the brink
And I need more ice
Ones that look like dice
Oh, I'll have a swim
(wish that I were trim)
Now I'm in the pool
Feeling quite a fool
Because I did forget
I don't like getting wet
I'll have another wine –
That one looks like mine
Wow! That's Chris's gin
My head's now in a spin
Whoops! I missed the seat –
Is that guy called Pete?
Musk have summore wine
Maybe he'sh called Brine?
Mush have a little nap an' more wine on tap
I'll just have 40 winksh
Then I'll hit the Linksh!

## PORTUGAL

Time I went to bed
Oh! A thumping head
Better take a paracetamol
(can't find anything to rhyme with paracetamol)!

Night Night!

# Soldier, Soldier

Soldier, soldier, sitting still,
While mosquitoes take their fill
No one knows that you are there
A statue in the still warm air
What you'd give to have a smoke,
Get in a bath and have a soak.
Don't even think about that beer
That you can almost taste from here.
You have important work to do
Keep watch until it's half past two
Don't make a move or scratch you're ear
The enemy will know you're here
You're playing an important role
The Exercise – that is your goal.
Don't think about your comfy bed
Sit up and rouse yourself instead
Focus on the "Hidden Eye"
If you can find it, it won't lie!

# tara

Young Tara at the breakfast table
Said "Eggs and Bacon, thank you Mable.
Make sure the eggs are freshly laid –
Oh, yes, I'd like some marmalade.
Toast and butter's just the thing
And when I want some more I'll ring"

Mable said "I've had enough"
And gave young Tara quite a cuff.
"I'm your Nanny, not your Slave
So, young lass will you behave.
Just sit and kindly wave a paw,
You lovely fat young Labrador".

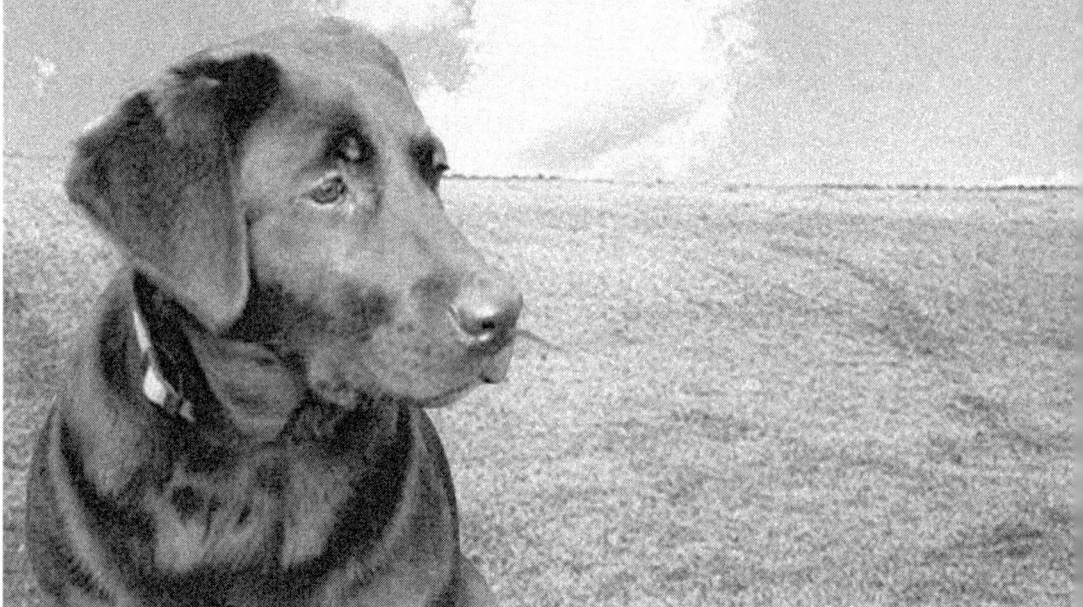

# THE CHRISTMAS FAIRY

When I grow up I want to be
A fairy on a Christmas tree
With baubles, lights and lots of glitter
My wand and wings would be a twitter.
Mummy says its not quite right
She thinks that I will look a sight
She worries what the neighbours think
And anyway I won't suit pink.
An Elf's outfit would be okay
Then that would make me just plain Gay!

# The Herberts

Once upon an olden time
Tansy wrote a little rhyme
The rhyme turned out to be a sonnet
That Tansy kept inside her bonnet.

Sometimes on the way to school
Tansy's friends would act the fool
They'd grab her bonnet off her head –
Replace it with some herbs instead

Her brother, Basil, was no help
Said he thought they could use kelp
But words won't stay within a weed
They need something that's grown from seed

They tried with Parsley, Dill and Sage
But still the words came off the page
The lesson of this simple rhyme
Is always keep a head of Thyme!

# THE PONY CLUB

The Pony Club is here again
They come in sleet and snow and rain
They come by road, some even trot
Most are smiling – some are not!
They come to hear how they must do it
But some will need a new "Round Touit"
With ponies strewn about the yard
The children learn and work quite hard
Which brushes are the best for what
And down a hill you must not trot!
I only hope they'll all remember
That lovely Friday last September
The sun shone down without a frown
Aren't we lucky not to live in a town.

# TIRAMISU

Tiramisu –
Say how do you do
To my tums and bums and thighs
I love you like crazy
But I am too lazy
To work out and so be wise
I'll eat till you're gone
Then there will be none
My waist will go up one size
I'll buy an O.S.
In a plain navy dress
And put up with my husband's sighs!

# VICTORIA PLUM

Oh, Victoria Plum
What have you done?
I'm afraid I love you lots.
I loved you in June
Which was far too soon
And now I've got the trots!

# When I was a dotty teenager

When I was young and in my teens
Ernie paid out – loads it seems.
I thought I'd spread my cash about
My brothers and their wives take out
But where to go – Ay, there's the rub –
No fun just going to the pub!
The Pony Club Ball – that seemed OK
And wasn't very far away
In Southport, at the Prince of Wales
An hotel that told many tales
We ate, we danced upon the table
And Don sang too, when he was able
I really can't remember a lot
I think somewhere I lost the plot
But one thing that sticks out by far
Was going home – 4 to a car,
Down Lord Street with horns a-blazing
It really was quite amazing.
With  Whoopee's and Talley-Ho's we go
Jan with her feet stuck out the window!

# OH BERNARD!

Oh Bernard my dear
You do look so queer
Do you think it was something you ate?
Your face is all green
Like a good runner bean
Not something you'd hang in the Tate.

I'll fetch you a bowl
A bucket and towel
I hope that I'll get there in time.
If you're going to be sick
Please do not pick –
What's that you're trying to mime?

Oh dear – I'm too late
Hang on for Pete's sake
I'm coming as fast as I can
Diced carrots again
It's always the same
Why can't you chuck up down the drain!

# THE CAT

I know you're a cat
A bright one at that
Why can't you remember the rule?
Mice and rats are OK
But at the end of the day,
Just one fish, not a whole school!

# THE FOOT OF MY STAIRS

Well I'll go to the foot of my stairs!

My Aunt said when life really glares.

I said "fancy that"

Aren't bungalows flat?

And as I recall

Have no stairs at all!

# HORSEY, HORSEY

Horsey, horsey, don't you buck
Just let your bum go hippity huk!
Your back is up
Your ears are down
Giddy up, we're homeward bound.

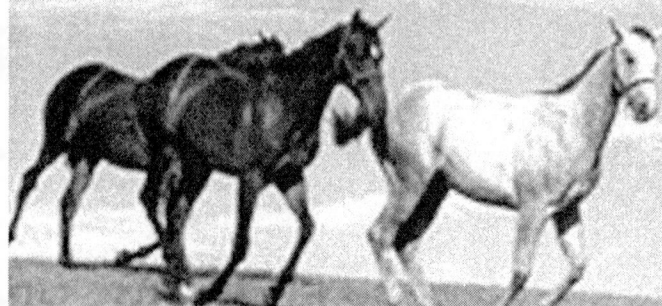

# A St. Georges Man

A St. George's man
That's what I am
I'm English through and through,
I wear a red cross
And don't give a toss
Of what others think I should do.

I've got an ambition
And loads of tuition
The Fusiliers now are my kin.
I now have a wife,
My trouble and strife
The rest of my life's just begin.

# ME (OR YOU?)

When I was young and in my prime
I misbehaved a lot of the time

There's stories that have got big lids
Any many things, not for kids

Like mushrooms they stay in the dark,
But when I tell them – what a lark!

They'll think that they're the only ones
That ever shook the bag of bones

Their parents never, never did
They don't think that that we could have hid

The fact that we have done before
The naughty bits that broke the law.

But the thing that worries me anon
Is what did our parents did for fun?

Maybe it is just as well
That, just like us, they did not tell.

Alli,
Mum, Second Mum, Adopted Mum,
Auntie Alli, Pal, Mate and Friend.

"You can shed tears that she is gone,
Or you can smile because she has lived.

You can close your eyes and pray that she shall come back,
Or you can open your eyes and see all that she has left.

Your heart can be empty because you can't see her,
Or you can be full of the love you shared.

You can turn your back on tomorrow and live yesterday,
Or you can be happy for tomorrow because of yesterday,

You can remember her and only that she has gone,
Or you can cherish her memory and let it live on.

You can cry and close your mind, be empty and turn your back,
Or you can do what she'd want – smile, open your eyes and go on."

An extract from Penny's dedication to Alli

The magic pencil writes,
And having written
It takes my breath away.
But as a born Britton,
I like the way words explode
Upon the virgin paper.
The shape, the sound, the mode,
What makes the words so clean,
Is when spoken sound sincere.

There will become a time
When poetry and rhyme
Will go totally out of my head
And instead of a stanza
There'll be a bonanza -
Perhaps it was something that I